MARINE'S P.T.

BOOT CAMP FITNESS

"You are what you do when nobody is watching"

-Darren Burch 2008

By Darren Burch

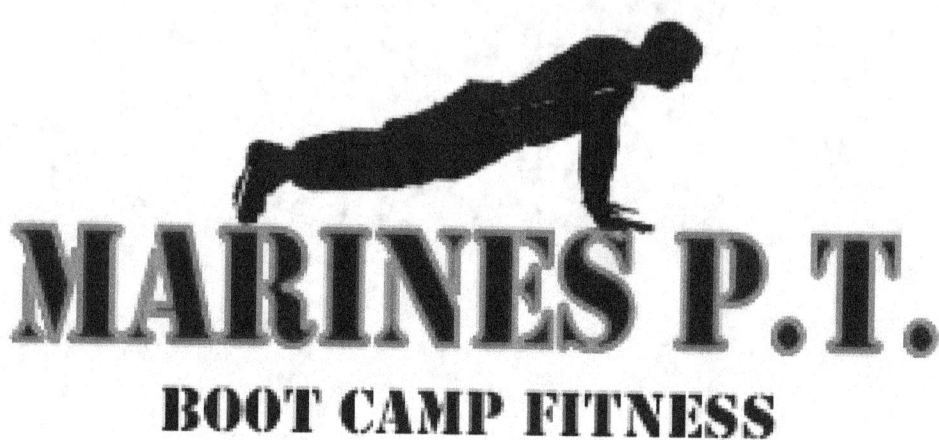

Created & Written by
Darren Burch

Photographed by
Adam Neal, C Marcelo Dube & Darren Burch

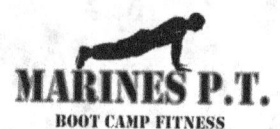

Marines P.T.
Boot Camp Fitness
Penguin Holdings LLC.
www.marinespt.com

The use of the words Marines P.T. are by no means to imply an endorsement, either implicit or explicit by the United Sates Marines Corps. Marines P.T. stands for Marine's possessive(me, I'm a former Marine Officer) and P.T. stands for Physical Training.

These exercises are the same or similar to what I experienced and used while serving in the United States Marine Corps. The names of the exercises and stretches are mostly common knowledge among Marines, but some exercise names and forms may be slightly modified or different than what is used in this book.

Please be advised to consult your physician before you conduct any strenuous exercise. I (the author) and Penguin Holdings LLC. disclaim any liability of injury resulting from the use of this exercise book. In other words, train and exercise at your own risk.

BULK ORDERS:
You can bulk order this book by contacting the author at:
marinespt@gmail.com

Cover designed by Darren Burch

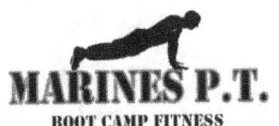

MARINES P.T.
BOOT CAMP FITNESS

DEDICATION

THIS BOOK IS DEDICATED TO MY TWO WONDERFUL CHILDREN,

SAMANTHA & DARREN II

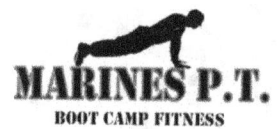

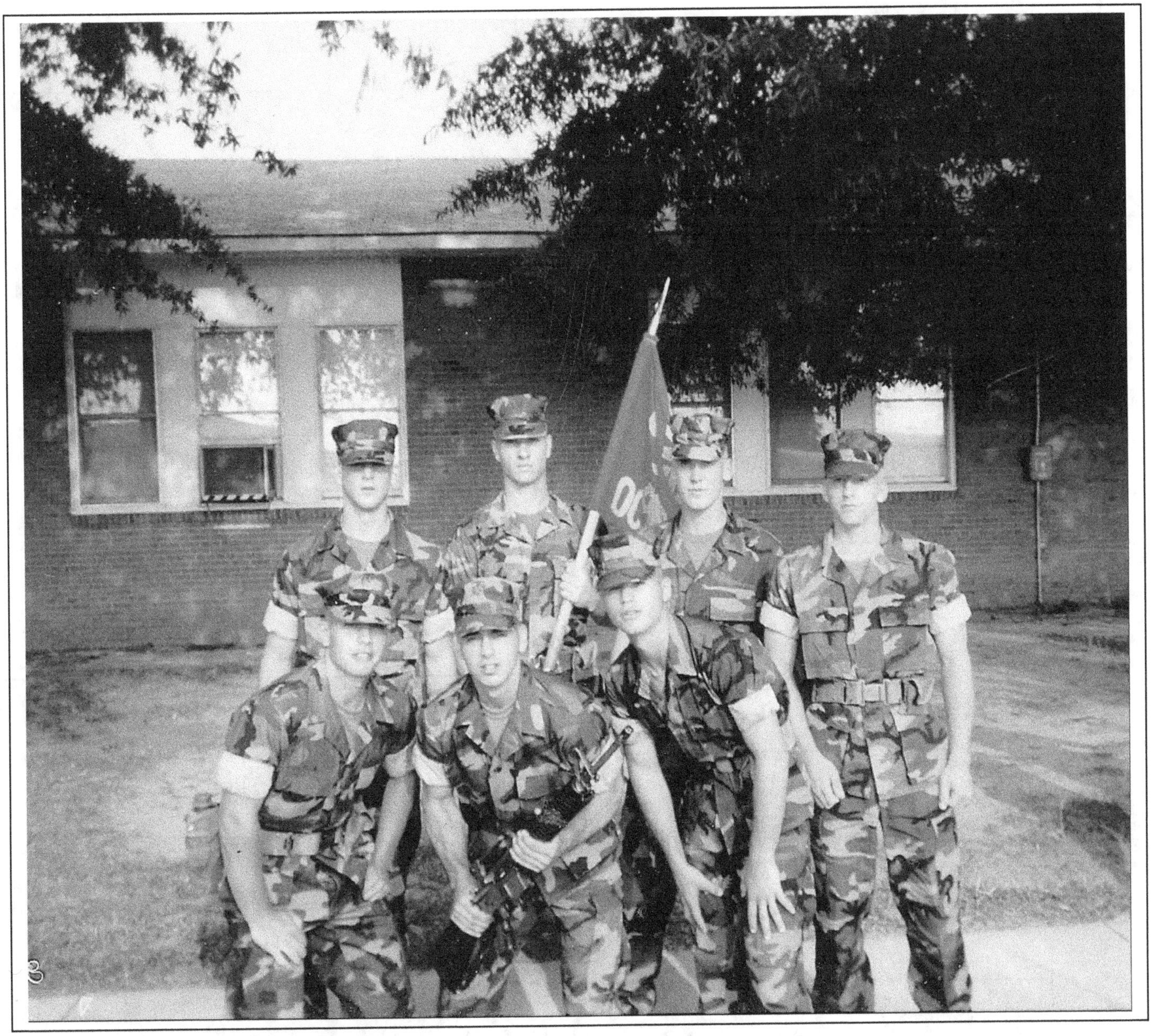

USMC Officer Candidate School (OCS) 1993.
These are all Aggies from Texas A&M University, and I'm the one with the rifle.

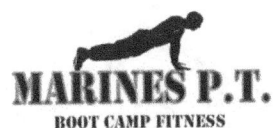

MARINES P.T.
BOOT CAMP FITNESS

TABLE OF CONTENTS

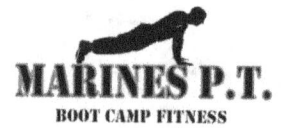

MARINES P.T.
BOOT CAMP FITNESS

PART I

INTRODUCTION

I have decided to put this book together to help more than just the people I come in contact with. This book is meant to be a book that you can pickup, select a workout, and take action. I did not intend to include "fluff" such as fitness philosophy, the history of fitness or any of the latest diet fads. I have also purposely left out lots of information on diet and nutrition. Diet and nutrition is a very personal subject and needs to be tailored to your body and your fitness goals. It could be an entire book by itself. I have read several fitness books and perused the bookshelves of major bookstores, looking for great workouts. All of them claim their program produces results, and for many of them I don't think that can be argued. I also found that it really depends on what kind of results you are looking for (i.e. Run time improvement, weight loss, cardio system improvement etc.) While I'm not going to make any such claims of guaranteed results, I will claim that the fitness program I use is all meat and no dessert. It has produced amazing and very significant physical results for my students. There are millions of fitness programs and nutritional tips out there, and many of them could work. The challenge is how much personal effort are <u>you</u> going to put into it? Fitness is a lifestyle and not a simple task that you move on from once you have met your goal. To actually achieve and sustain the fitness results you want, you can <u>never stop</u>, and you can never give up!

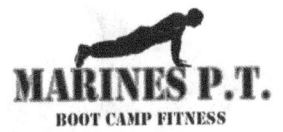

BIO

(Condensed and fast forwarded)

I grew up in the town of Webster, TX. It was a small bedroom community just south of Houston, TX that along with Clear Lake, TX housed many of the NASA engineers and employees. I played sports in high school (football, basketball, and track) and always kept very active. High School was a blur. . I worked at fast food, and then moved up to retail selling shoes to pay for car insurance and dates with my girlfriend. I made mostly A's and took a few honors classes. Luckily, I did well enough to get accepted to a great college, Texas A&M. I then found myself in the Corps of Cadets at Texas A&M University, and going through quite the transformation. I won't bore you too much in this book about my experience in the Corps of Cadets. Suffice it to say that I started with 27 freshman buddies and only 10 of us made it through our freshman year. So fast forwarding… After graduating from Texas A&M with a degree in Political Science, I was commissioned a 2nd Lieutenant in the United Stated Marine Corps.

As I write this, I can think of enough stories from my college years and time in the Marines for a completely separate book. There was plenty of victory, fun, sadness, fear, love, growing up, tons of comedy, craziness and perseverance…but I digress. I spent six years in the Marines. Three of them were as an Artillery Officer that included a 6-month deployment to the Mediterranean (many stories here…including inebriated Marines singing karaoke in Malta for my birthday. My final 2 ½ years were spent at the Marine

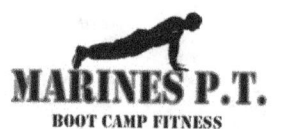

Corps Recruit Depot (MCRD) "Boot Camp", in San Diego, California, which is what ties all of this together.

My time at MCRD is arguably some of the best times of my life. It was there that I could witness the amazing transformation of young men and women right off the block into lean mean fighting machines, They became United States Marines. What the Marine Corps can do in just 13 weeks would rival the best efforts of any successful company in the world. That kind of accomplishment instilled a great sense of pride and honor in these new young Marines and being a part of it changed me forever.

While training new Marine recruits I competed in triathlons in San Diego, and a crazy 200 mile, 12 hour, mountainous bike ride in Davis, California called the Davis Double Century. Fitness for me was already a lifestyle I just didn't know it. Fast forwarding…. I left the Marines in 2000 to go to work for IBM in Silicon Valley. I had two awesome kiddos along the way (Samantha & Darren II the joys of my life) and came back to Texas to work for Home Depot as a store manager. It was at Home Depot that I earned my stripes in retail. I enjoyed Home Depot but I found a better opportunity with Target, and began working for them as a store manager. Fast forwarding again…. I was promoted with Target to district manager, and in 2008 I decided to pursue fitness as a business, and started Marines P.T. Boot Camp Fitness. There are many stories in between, but that's for another time. Many of my experiences further instilled a sense of drive and perseverance inside of me that keeps me saying NEVER GIVE UP!

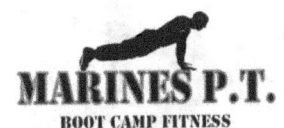

MARINES P.T.

BOOT CAMP FITNESS

The exercises I use in my boot camp program are mostly based on the very same exercises I used while in the Marines. There are 16 workout sessions for you to use consecutively. You can, and probably will, modify these workouts to suit your goals, but try to complete them as I have them here.

Each workout session includes a stretching and exercise group that I describe in the next few pages. After completing the warm up, stretching and exercise groups, there is a "main event" workout to complete the session. In some sessions you will need to complete an additional exercise group after the "main event". There are also photos of the correct form for each exercise at the end of the book.

If you put forth the highest effort you can during each exercise, and use the correct form, you will get what you are after, RESULTS. I certainly don't want any delusions of grandeur that this is the silver bullet of fitness. It takes great personal effort, proper diet, and perseverance, to win and achieve your fitness goals. So get to it.

Here are a few of my favorite famous USMC quotes to help get you in the mindset.

USMC quotes:

"Sometimes it is entirely appropriate to kill a fly with a sledge-hammer!" Major Holdredge.

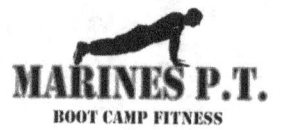

"The safest place in Korea was right behind a platoon of Marines. Lord, how they could fight!"

"Panic sweeps my men when they are facing the American Marines." Captured North Korean Major.

"Some people spend an entire lifetime wondering if they made a difference. The Marines don't have that problem." President Ronald Reagan.

"Casualties many; Percentage of dead not known; Combat efficiency: We are winning!" Colonel David M. Shoup, USMC

"So they've got us surrounded. Good. That simplifies the problem! Now we can fire in any direction, those bastards won't get away this time!" Chesty Puller, USMC, during the forgotten Korean War.

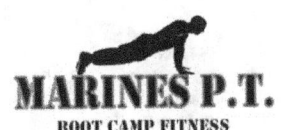

PART II

The Warm Up, Stretching & Exercise Groups

These are the different warm up, stretching, and exercise groups I refer to in each of my 19 workout sessions. In every session I use at a minimum 1 stretching group and 1 exercise group. After the first few sessions I eliminate the warm up, but **NEVER** skip the stretching. In the Marines we called these our daily 16. The daily 16 consist of 8 stretches and 8 callisthenic exercises done before the "main event".

WARM UP GROUP

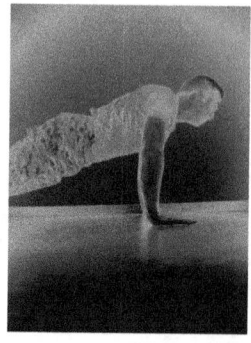

> * **START** running in place
>   Punch fists to front
>   Punch fists upward
>   Arm circles
> * **END** running in place
>   Neck **ROTATIONS**
>   Knee & ankle rotations
>   Waist rotations.

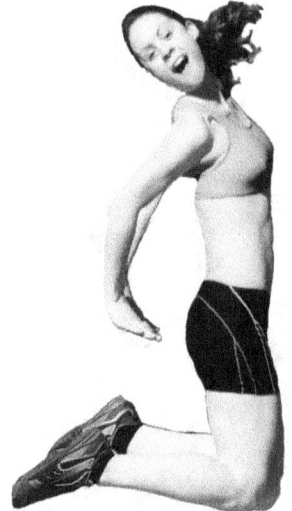

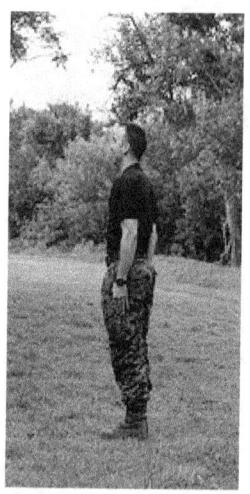

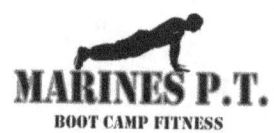

MARINES P.T.
BOOT CAMP FITNESS

STRETCHING GROUPS

STRETCHING GROUP 1
TRICEPS STRETCH
CHEST STRETCH
CALF STRETCH
SHOULDER STRETCH
HIP & BACK HOLLYWOODS
QUAD STRETCH
HAMSTRING STRETCH
GROIN STRETCH

STRETCHING GROUP 2
TRICEPS STRETCH
SHOULDER STRETCH
CHEST STRETCH
CALF STRETCH
MODIFIED HURDLER STRETCH
ITB STRETCH LYING
QUAD STRETCH
GROIN STRETCH

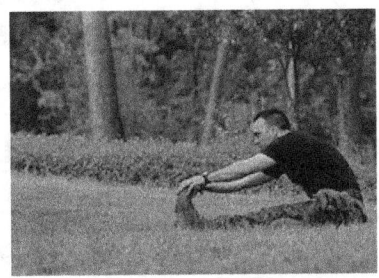

STRETCHING GROUP 3
TRICEPS STRETCH
SHOULDER STRETCH
CHEST STRETCH
CALF STRETCH
MODIFIED HURDLER STRETCH
HOLLYWOODS
QUAD STRETCH
GROIN STRETCH

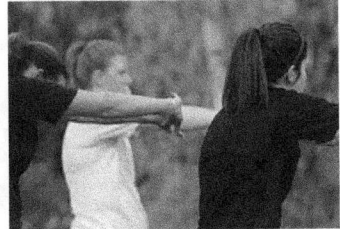

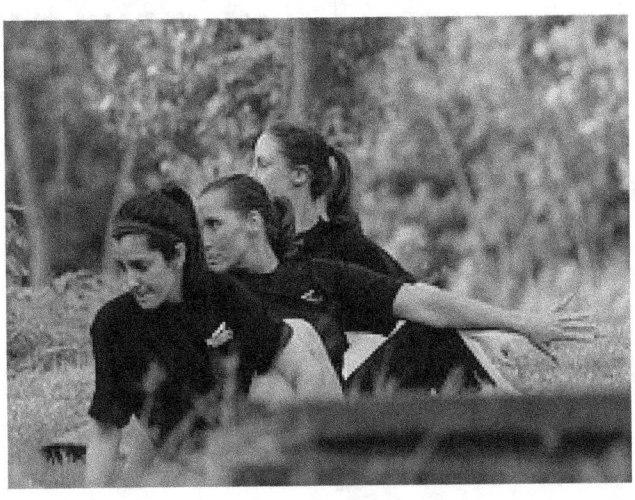

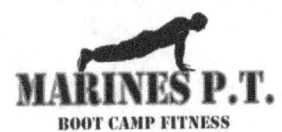

MARINES P.T.
BOOT CAMP FITNESS

EXERCISE GROUPS

**ALL EXERCISES ARE DONE IN 4 COUNTS. THE NUMBERS IN PARENTHESES ARE THE NUMBER OF 4 COUNT REPETITIONS.

EXERCISE GROUP 1
SIDE STRADDLE HOPS (20)
PUSH UPS (10)
SIDE CRUNCHES (15)
FLUTTER KICKS (15)
DIRTY DOGS (15)
DONKEY KICKS (15)
ELBOW TO KNEE CRUNCHES (15)
STEAM ENGINES (15)

EXERCISE GROUP 2
SIDE STRADDLE HOPS (20)
8 COUNT BODY BUILDERS (12)
WIDE ANGLE PUSHUPS (10)
CRUNCHES (15)
MOUNTAIN CLIMBERS (20)
LUNGES (15)
PUSH UPS (10)
DIVE BOMBER PUSHUPS (15)

EXERCISE GROUP 3
SIDE STRADDLE HOPS (25)
FLUTTER KICKS (20)
WIDE ANGLE PUSHUPS (10)
CRUNCHES (20)
MOUNTAIN CLIMBERS (20)
SIDE CRUNCHES (15)
STEAM ENGINES (20)
LUNGES (15)

EXERCISE GROUP 4
SIDE STRADDLE HOPS (30)
8 COUNT BODY BUILDERS (12)
PUSHUPS (12)
CRUNCHES (20)
DIRTY DOGS (20)
DONKEY KICKS (20)
FLUTTER KICKS (20)
MOUNTAIN CLIMBERS (20)

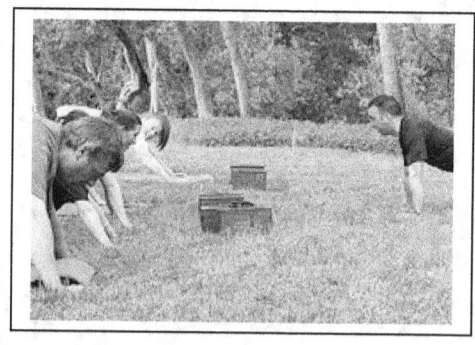

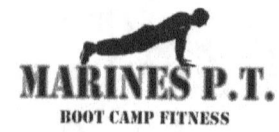

MARINES P.T.
BOOT CAMP FITNESS

PART III

EXERCISE SESSIONS

Each session is about 45 to 55 minutes long. Remember to only do as many repetitions as you can complete with good form. Start with session 1 and progress your way to session 19. Read all the sessions before you start the first one. You will need to make sure you have a great place to do these workout sessions. I recommend you do 3 to 5 sessions per week. Once you reach the final session congratulate yourself. Then start over and increase all your reps by at least 5. One suggestion: Make copies of the Warm-up, Stretch, and Exercise pages out of this book, then laminate them and cut out each card group to carry with you.

I also recommend that you do the sessions with breaks between sessions. I do sessions on Monday, Wednesday, Thursday, and Saturday. This gives your body a chance to recover.

GOOD LUCK!

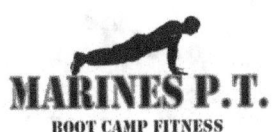

MARINES P.T.
BOOT CAMP FITNESS

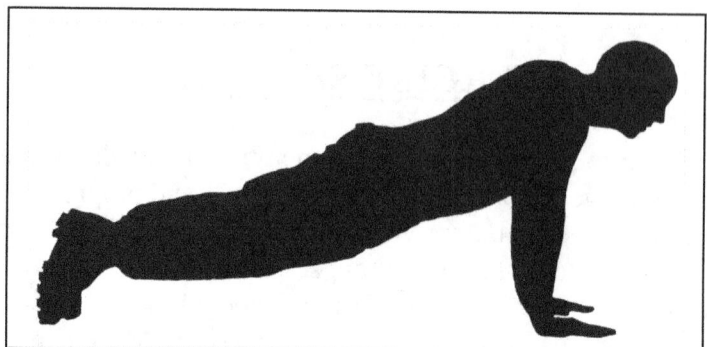

SESSION 1:
Weigh-in, Warm-up group, Stretch group 1, Inventory PFT (1.5 mile run, total pushups in 2 minutes, total crunches in 2 minutes) Stretch group 1. PFT stands for Physical Fitness Test. Start with a fitness test so you can measure progress. Record your weight. If you have a fancy scale that records body fat, then record that too.

- PFT Push-ups: make sure the person does a proper push-up as demonstrated in this book
- PFT Crunches: The crunches for the PFT are Marine Corps standard crunches. You will need someone to hold your feet to the ground.
- <u>**Take note: This is not the USMC fitness test. You should include a 3 mile run and pull-ups or flex arm hang into your workouts if you are preparing for boot camp. I have made some suggestions in each session where you can include pull-ups and longer runs for your PFT.**</u>

SESSION 2:
Warm-up, Stretch group 2, Exercise group 1, **Ammo can steps**, 20 minute run 80% of max pace(should be a fast jog). Exercise group 2.

- **Ammo cans** – I use 7.62mm ammo cans with a 1 gallon Ziploc bag filled with sand. They weigh about 8lbs each. You can substitute dumbbells, but think about how cool it looks to use ammo cans.
- <u>**The ammo can steps**</u> is an exercises that you run up 2 or 3 steps and backwards that same 2 or 3 steps as fast as you can and staying on your toes for 1 minute. You then rest for 1 minute, then go again for 4 sets.

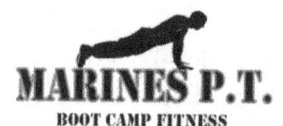

MARINES P.T.
BOOT CAMP FITNESS

SESSION 3: Stretch group 2, Exercise group 3, **Circuit Course** 20 min (5-8 stations), Stretch group 2.

- **Circuit Course:** This is essentially a session where you run from station to station to complete and exercises for 1 minute at each station. Select one of the 4 exercises cards to use as a guide if needed. I like 2 or 4 for this. You will need to be creative depending on where you are working out. I use some plastic signs placed in the ground to set up the course throughout the park. However, you don't have to have signs…just do the exercises after running for about 2 to 3 minutes.

SESSION 4: Stretch group 3 & Exercise group 3, 2 mile timed run (3 mile time run for those going into boot camp), Exercise group 4 (sub **pull-up pyramid** for the exercise group 4 if you are going to boot camp), stretch group 3.

- On your 2 mile run, you should run at 85-90% of your max pace.
- **Pull-up Pyramid:** This will vary depending on how may pull-ups you can do. Start with doing 4 pull-ups then go to 5, then 6, then 7, then 7, 6, 5, 4. Adjust these up or down depending on your ability. You goal should be to do 20 dead hang pull-ups. This will help you score big on your USMC PFT.

SESSION 5: Stretch group 1 & Exercise group 1, **Ammo can lunges**, **Indian run** 20 minutes, Stretch 1 & Exercise groups 1 – intro to **16 count body builders** – do 10 o of the 16 count body builders.

- **Ammo can lunges:** take your ammo cans or weights and do the lunges exercise. You should to 3 sets (15, 12, then 10 repetitions). Increase, as you get stronger.
- **Indian run:** Line up with your group in a single file line. Begin a slow jog pace with everyone spread out about 10 feet or more. Then the person at the very back of the line sprints to the front. Once the person from the rear makes it to the front and settles into the jog pace, the next person from the rear sprints to the front. This works best if you have 4 or more people.
- **16 count body builders**: Just like 8 count body builders but instead you open and close your legs three times, then do three pushups…all before you come back up for a total of 16 counts.

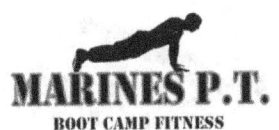

MARINES P.T.
BOOT CAMP FITNESS

SESSION 6: Stretch 3 & Exercise group 4, **Log drills 4x6 log**, **Ammo can sprints/races**, Stretch group 2.

- **Log Drills:** At Boot Camp we had a long log/pole for as many as 10 recruits to pick up and run with, or do sit-ups with all together. What I use at my Boot Camp is a 4"x6" log about 2 feet long bought from a lumberyard or home improvement store. Do 3 sets of overhead log lifts, going from one shoulder, over your head, and to the other shoulder. Then do 3 sets of crunches, holding the log across your stomach. Touch your knees with the log for each crunch.
- **Ammo can sprints/races:** These will vary depending on where you are working out and what is available to you. I use a very big hill because it's available to me…much to the pain of my students. The intent is to run for about 100 yards with the ammo cans put them down, run back to your starting point, then run back and grab the ammo cans and bring them back to your starting point. That completes one set. You can race each other if you have a group. Do 4 sets of these sprint races. My students tell me this is one of the toughest workouts, and I must admit, if you put out it's pretty darn tough. Hills work best here. So if you can find a good hill, it's a race to the top and back down.

SESSION 7: Stretch & Exercise group 2, **Circuit Course** 25 min, slow run 10 minutes cool down, stretch group 2. (add 3 sets of 8 pull-ups for USMC PFT)
- Do the circuit course as described in session 3 but spend 1-½ minutes at each station.

SESSION 8: Stretch 1 & Exercise group 1, Ammo can lunges drill, **crunches galore!** 12 count body builders, Stretch group 1 (Abs stretch. See demo photo).

- **Crunches galore:** Do 3 sets of 25 crunches. All are 4 count (or do 3 sets of 100 crunches.)
- **Ammo Can Lunges:** Do the same lunges as described in session 5. Try to increase to 4 sets (15, 12, 12, 10)
- Do 3 sets of 12 count body builders (10, 10, 10)

SESSION 9: Stretch 3 & Exercise group 4, ammo cans steps 1-½ minutes 3 sets, Indian run 22 minutes, Stretch Group 3 (add pull-up pyramid for USMC PFT)

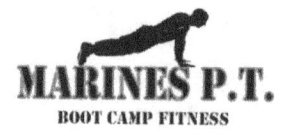

SESSION 10: Stretch Group 2, mid PFT, Stretch group 2.

- This is good time to take a Physical Fitness Test (PFT) to see how you are doing. Record your push-ups, sit-ups, and 1.5 mile run time. Sub pull-ups for push-ups and make the run a 3 mile run if you are taking the USMC PFT.

SESSION 11: Stretch 1 & Exercise group 4; log drills 4x6 log, 2-mile run, stretch group 1.

SESSION 12: Stretch 2 & Exercise group 2, Crunches Galore! medium paced run 20 minutes at 75% max pace, Exercise group 4. (sub pull-up pyramid)

SESSION 13: Stretch & Exercise group 1, **Mini circuit course** 15 minutes include steps or stairs, pushups x10, crunches x40. 2 mile run ability pace.

- **Mini Circuit Course:** This is done just like the regular circuit course but you should only do 4 or 5 stations and no need to set up signs for this one. I include running up some hills and stairs in this one as well as a set of push-ups and crunches at the end. Sub pull-ups if you can for USMC PFT.

SESSION 14: Stretch 3 & Exercise group 3, Ammo can steps(3 sets), Ammo can sprints/races(4 sets). Stretch group 3.

SESSION 15: Stretch 1 & Exercise group 4, taper- slow 3-mile run, stretch 1

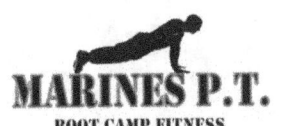

MARINES P.T.
BOOT CAMP FITNESS

SESSION 16: Stretch group 3, **Final PFT** (1.5 mile run, pushups in 2 minutes, crunches in 2 minutes). Replace the 1.5 mile run with the 3 mile run, and the push-ups with pull-ups for USMC PFT. GO ALL OUT 100% EFFORT!

SESSION 17: Stretch group 2, Exercise group 2, Change-up run (Jog 2 minutes, sprint 45 seconds. Repeat for 20 minutes total)

SESSION 18: Stretch 3 & Exercise group 3, **Steps run** 24 minutes. (Run stairs everywhere in park)
- **Steps run:** You can incorporate stairs into your run on this one. This is going to depend on what you have to work with at the place you workout. You can also do stadium bleachers if you have access to one.

SESSION 19: Stretch group 1 & Exercise group 4. Mini circuit course for 17 minutes. Run and stop where you want to do an exercise (Instructor's discretion). Stretch group 3 afterwards.

YOU MADE IT!!
CONGRATS!!

Now go back to session 1 and increase your reps!
Move it! Move it!

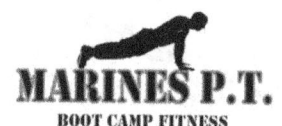

MARINES P.T.
BOOT CAMP FITNESS

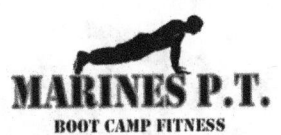

WARM UP DEMO PHOTOS

These warm-up exercises are all conducted while running.

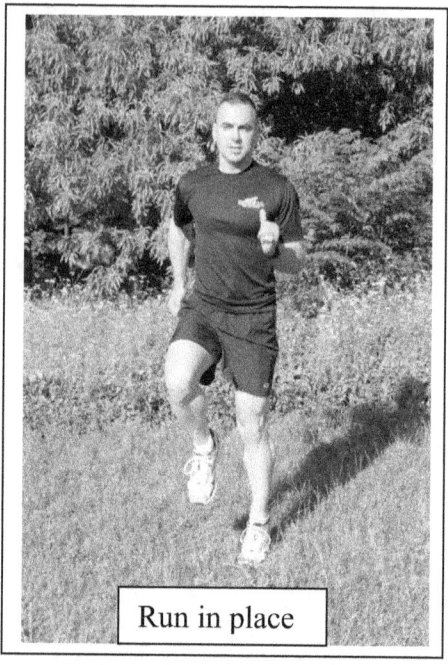

Run in place

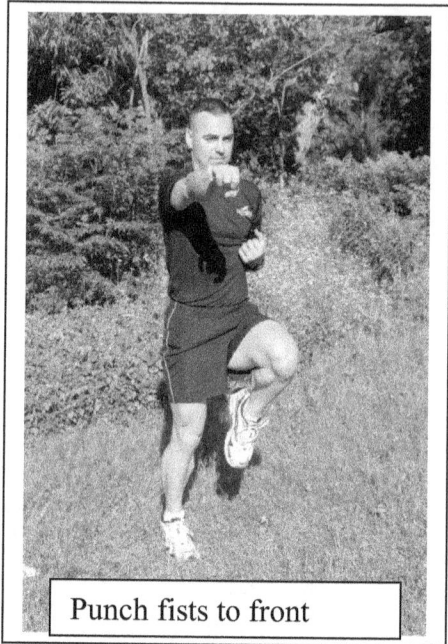

Punch fists to front

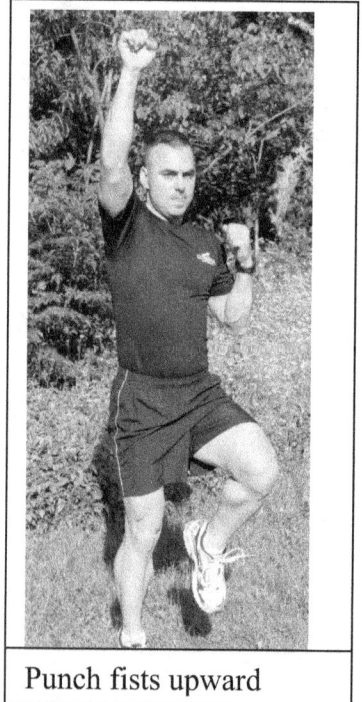

Punch fists upward

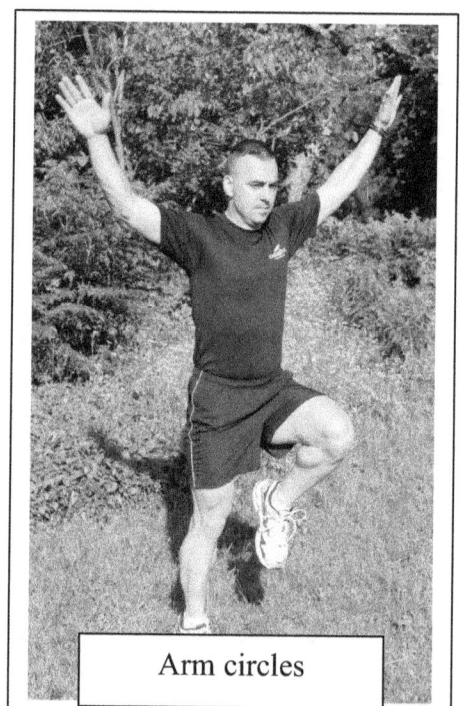

Arm circles

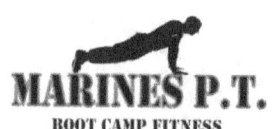

MARINES P.T.
BOOT CAMP FITNESS

NECK ROTATION

Standing in place roll your neck from front to side to back.

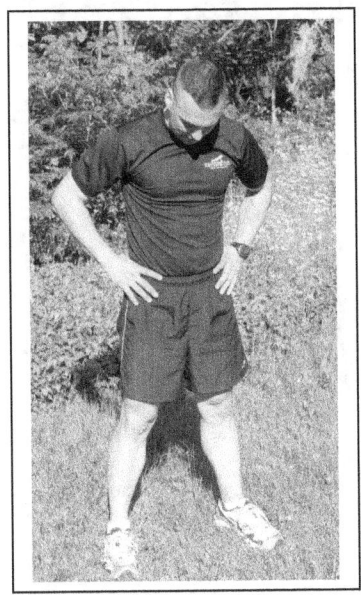
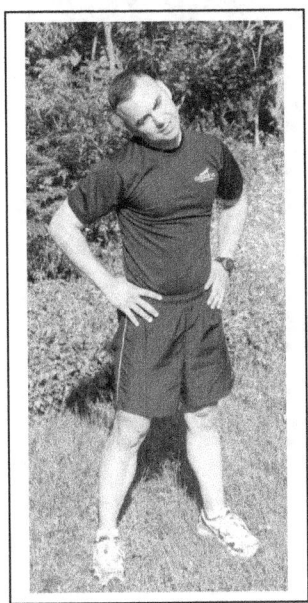

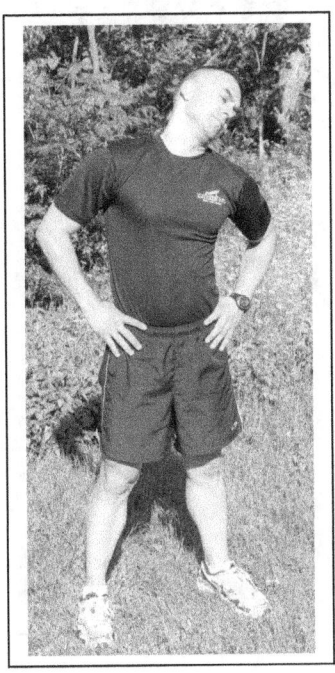

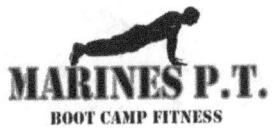

MARINES P.T.
BOOT CAMP FITNESS

KNEE ROTATION

Standing in place roll your knees from front to side to back.

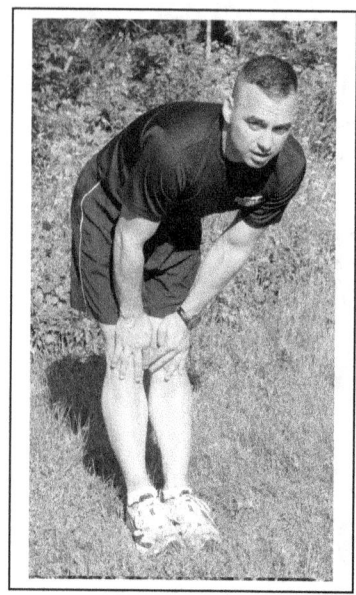 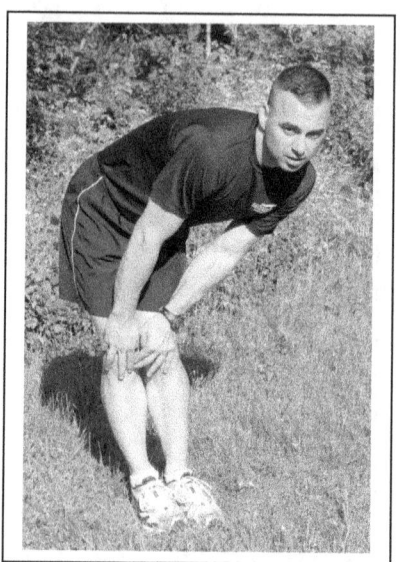

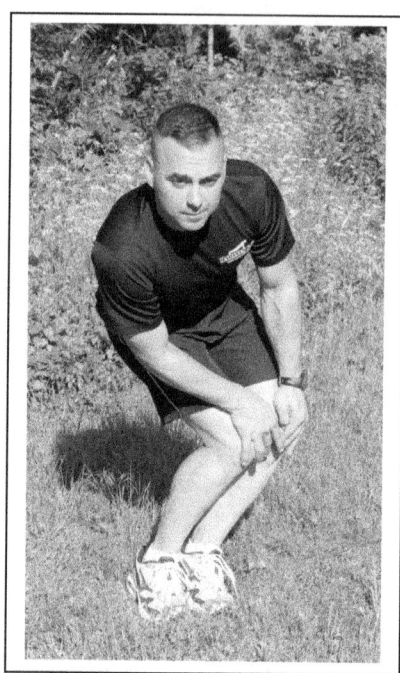

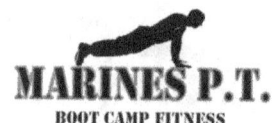

STRETCHING DEMO PHOTOS

TRICEPS STRETCH

- Place your hand in the small of your back and pull back on the elbow to stretch your triceps. Repeat with each arm for a count of 10.

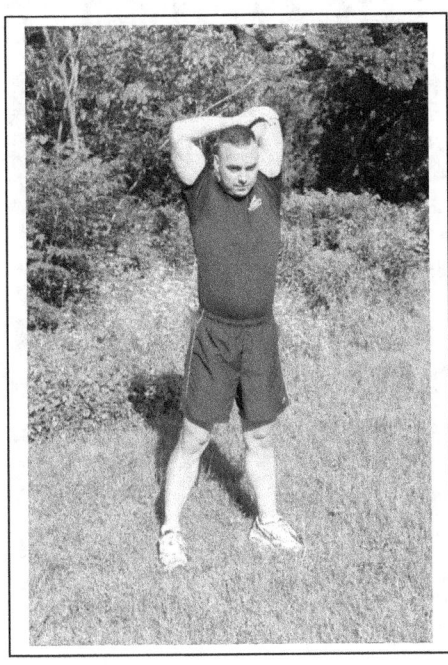
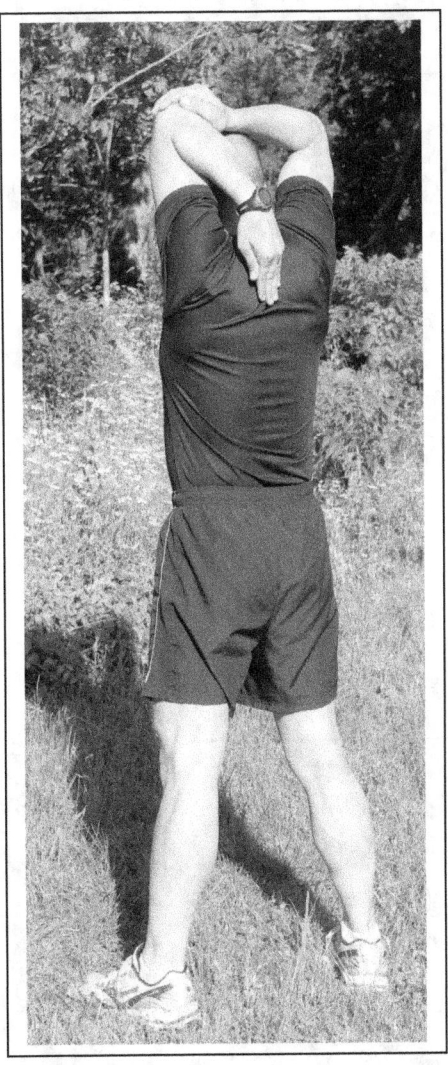

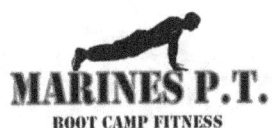

MARINES P.T.
BOOT CAMP FITNESS

BACK & SHOULDER STRETCH

Clasp your hands together and push forward to stretch your back and shoulders.

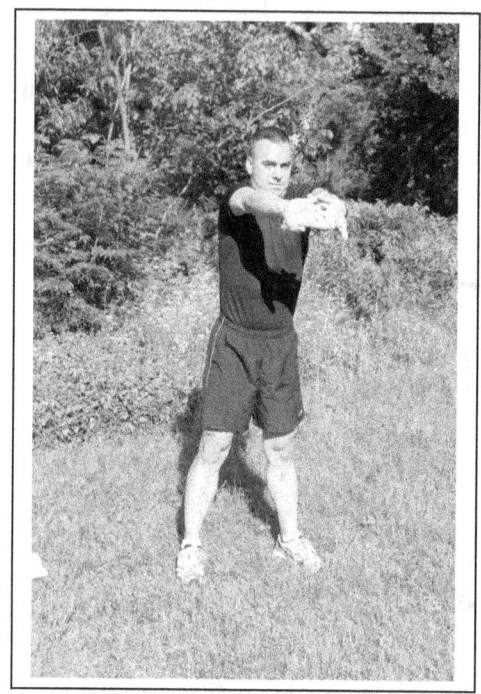

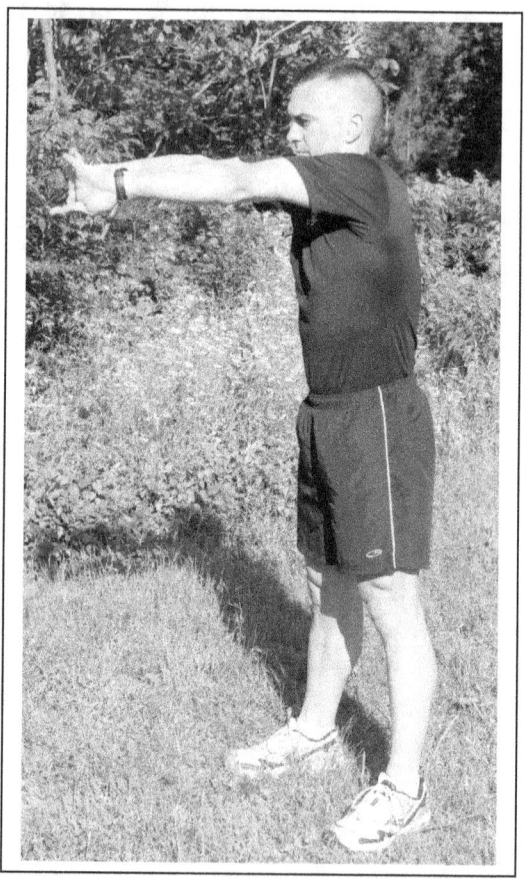

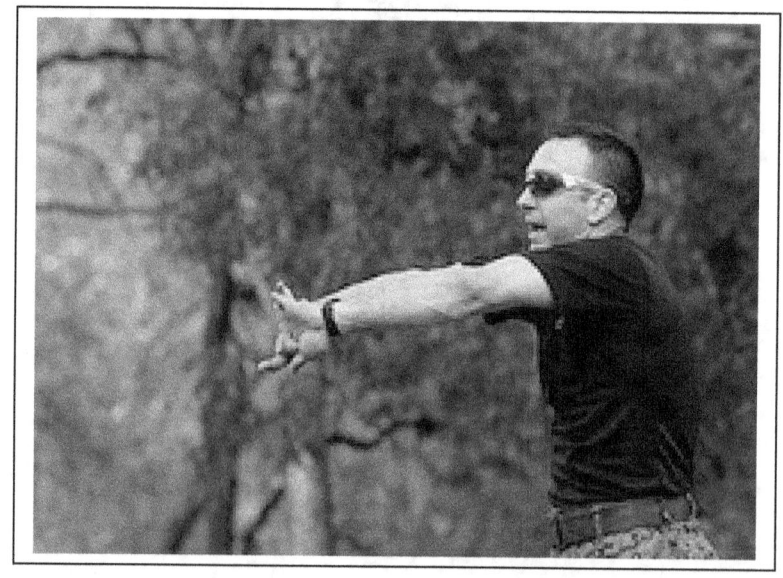

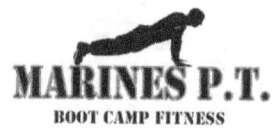

MARINES P.T.
BOOT CAMP FITNESS

CHEST STRETCH

Clasp your hands together behind you and push upward with your arms to stretch your chest.

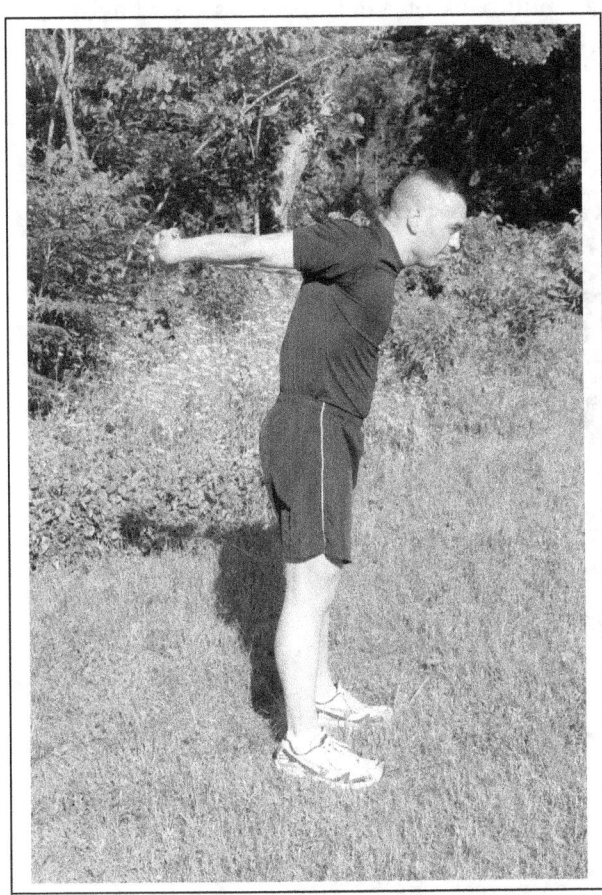

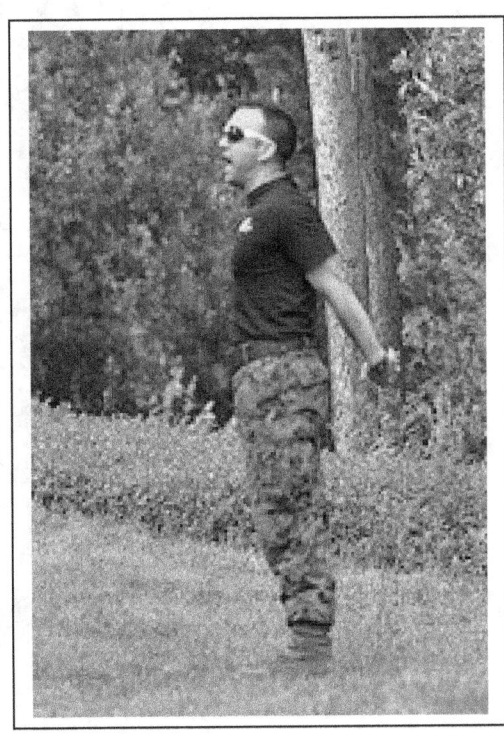

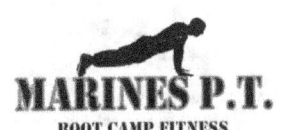

MARINES P.T.
BOOT CAMP FITNESS

CALF STRETCH

Place your right heel into the ground as shown and bend your left leg. Place your weight mostly on your left leg, and while bending down pull back on your toes with your hand. You should feel the flex and pull of the calf. Repeat this process with your left leg.

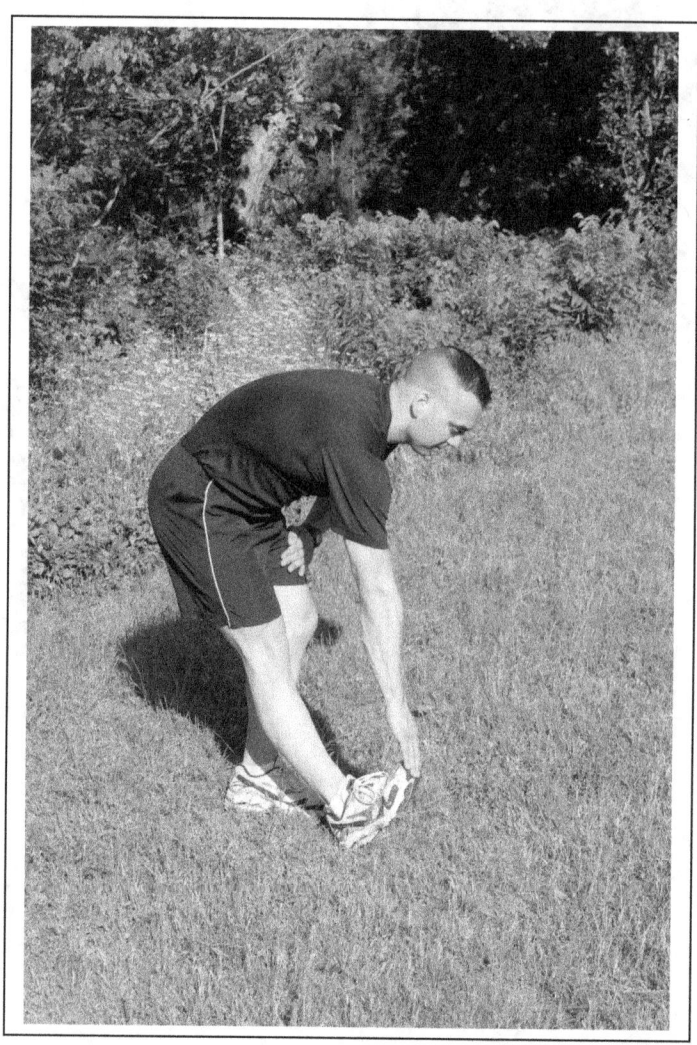

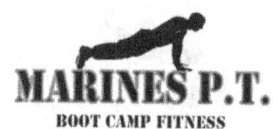

MARINES P.T.
BOOT CAMP FITNESS

HOLLYWOODS
(Also called a hip and back stretch)

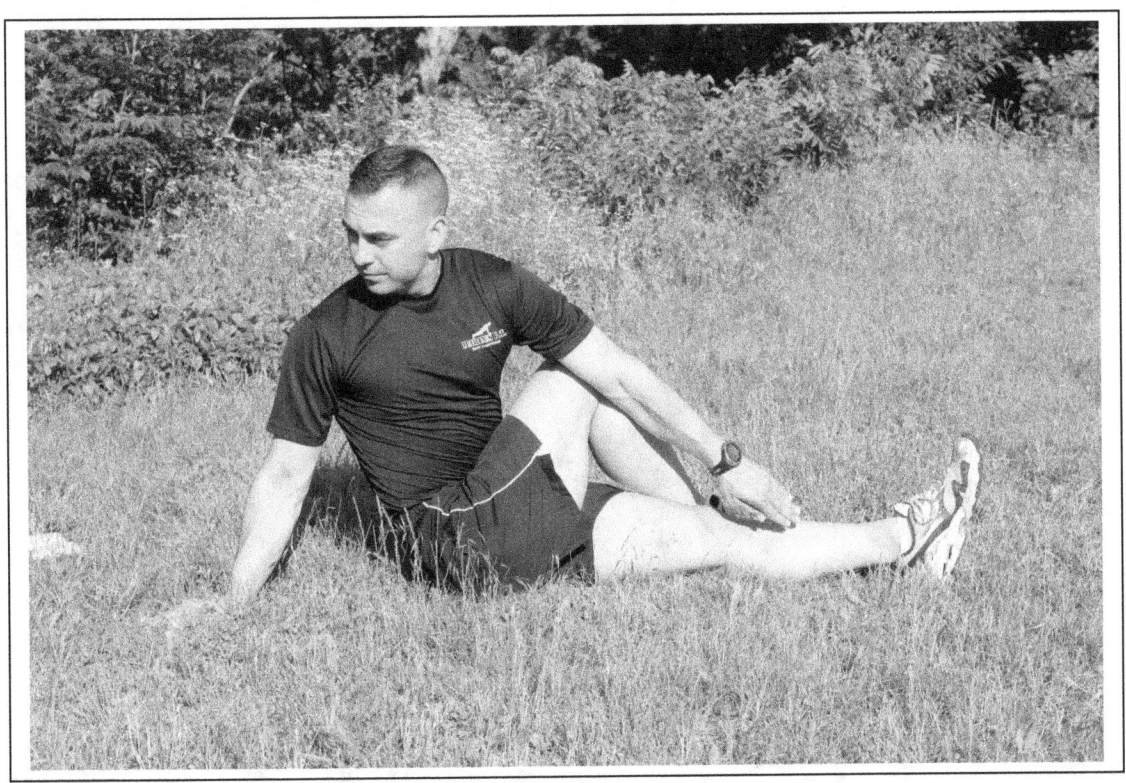

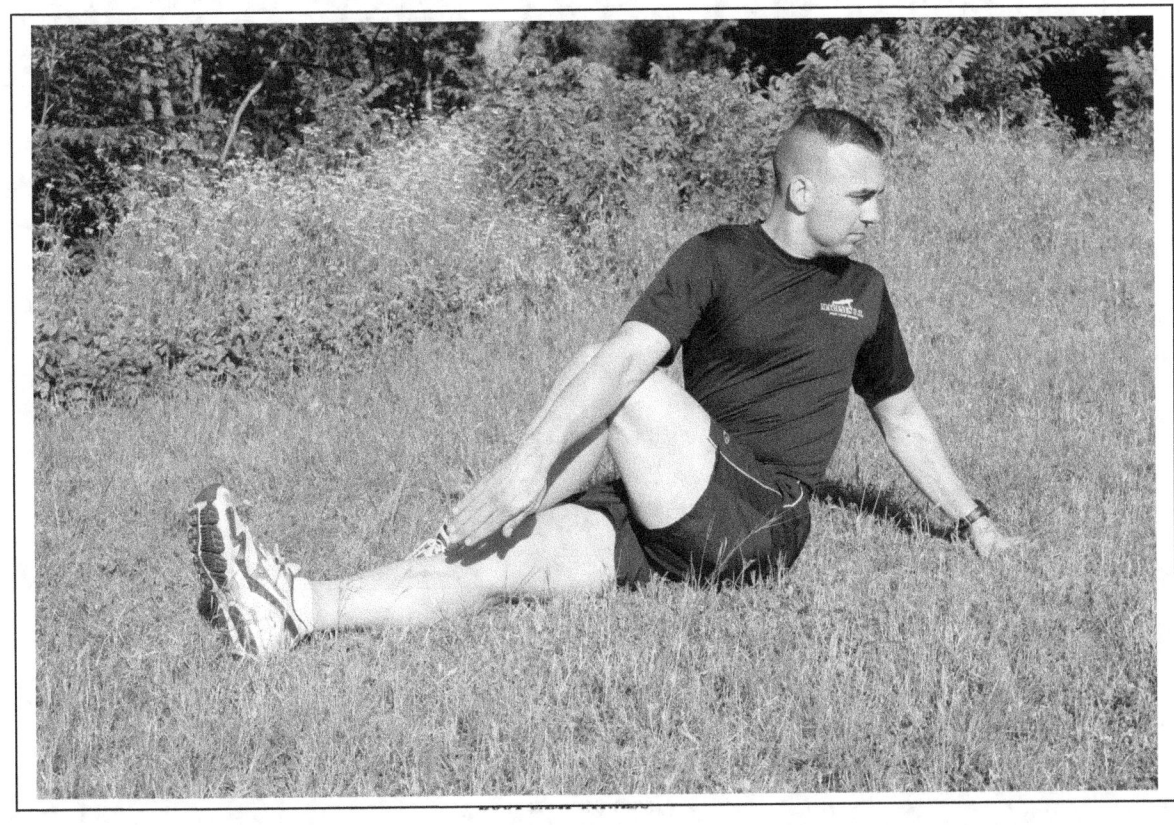

HURDLER STRETCH MODIFIED

Tuck your right leg into your left thigh tightly. Make sure you keep your left knee straight. Grab or touch your toes with BOTH hands as shown below. This mostly stretches your hamstrings. Repeat for the other leg.

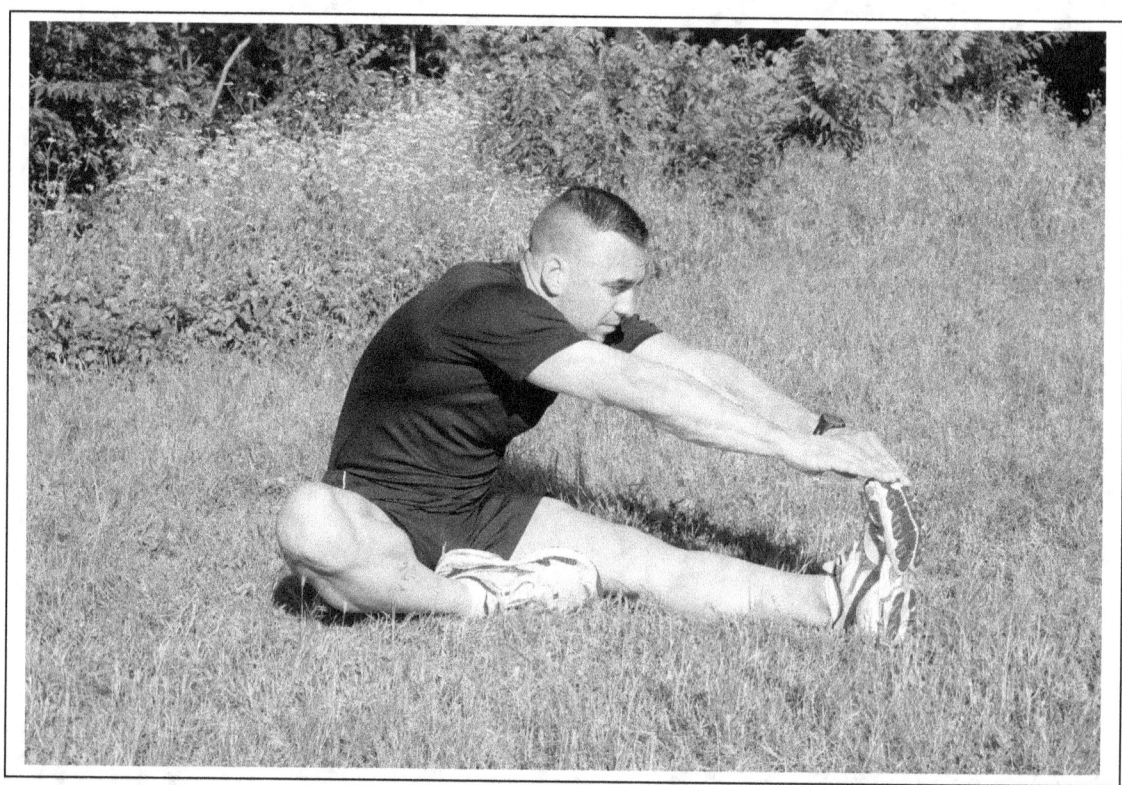

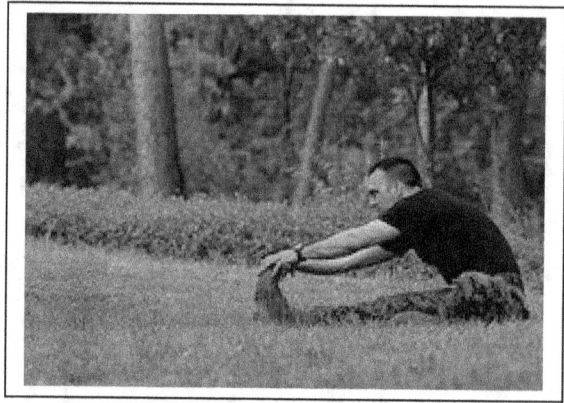

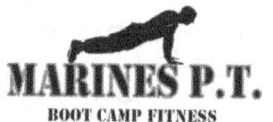

MARINES P.T.
BOOT CAMP FITNESS

ITB STRETCH

Lying on your back, pull your right leg upward from behind your knee while bent 90 degrees. Use your right hand (not shown) to stabilize yourself.

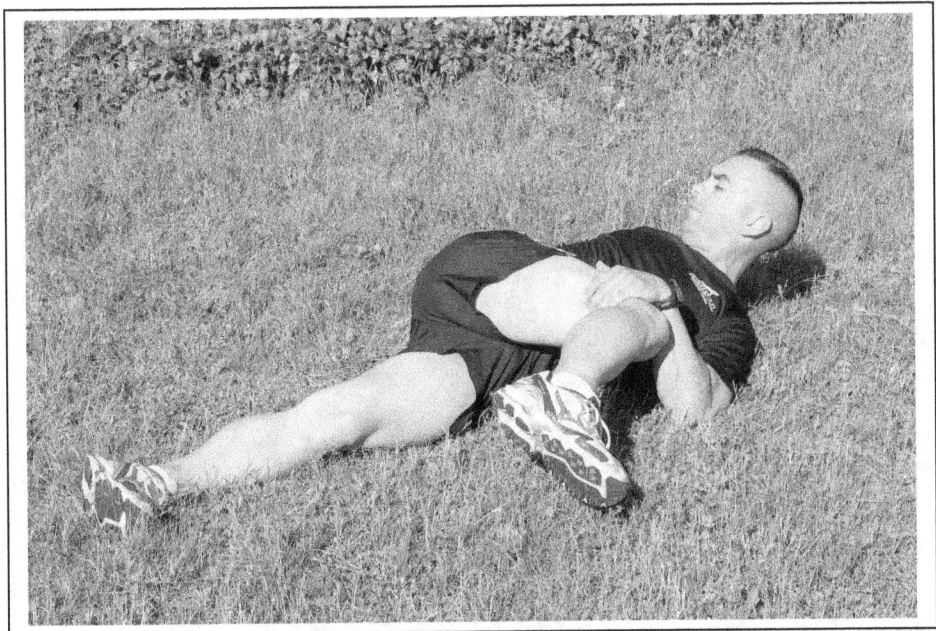

GROIN STRETCH

Bring your heels into your groin and grab your ankles. Press downward on your knees to try and push them to the ground with your elbows.

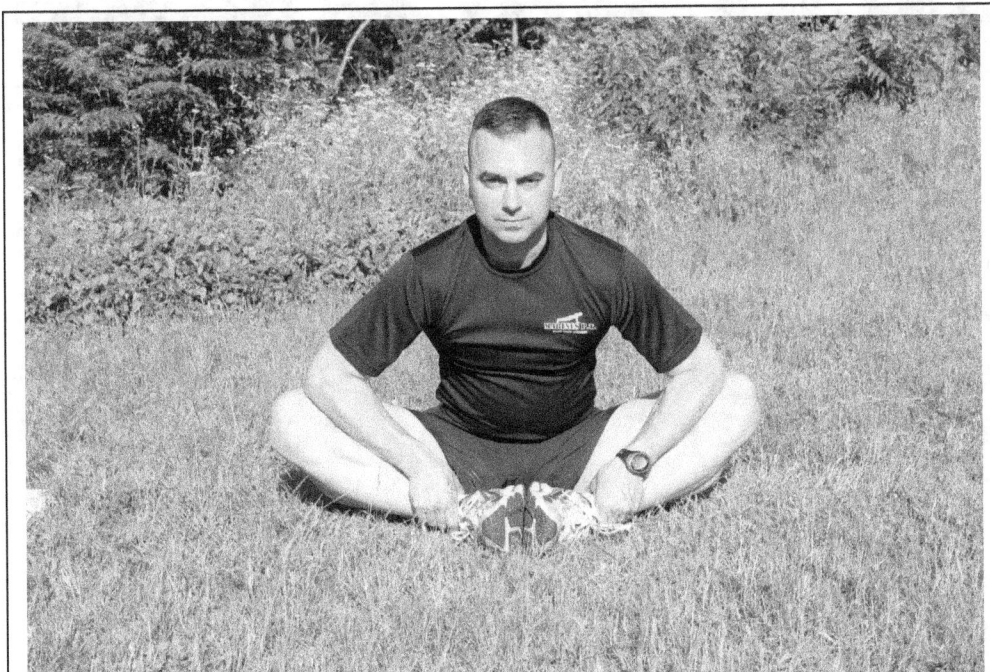

QUAD STRETCH

Lying on your left side, pull your right foot back such that your right heel touches your rear, and your right knee goes slightly backward. Repeat with your left leg. You can also do this stretch standing.

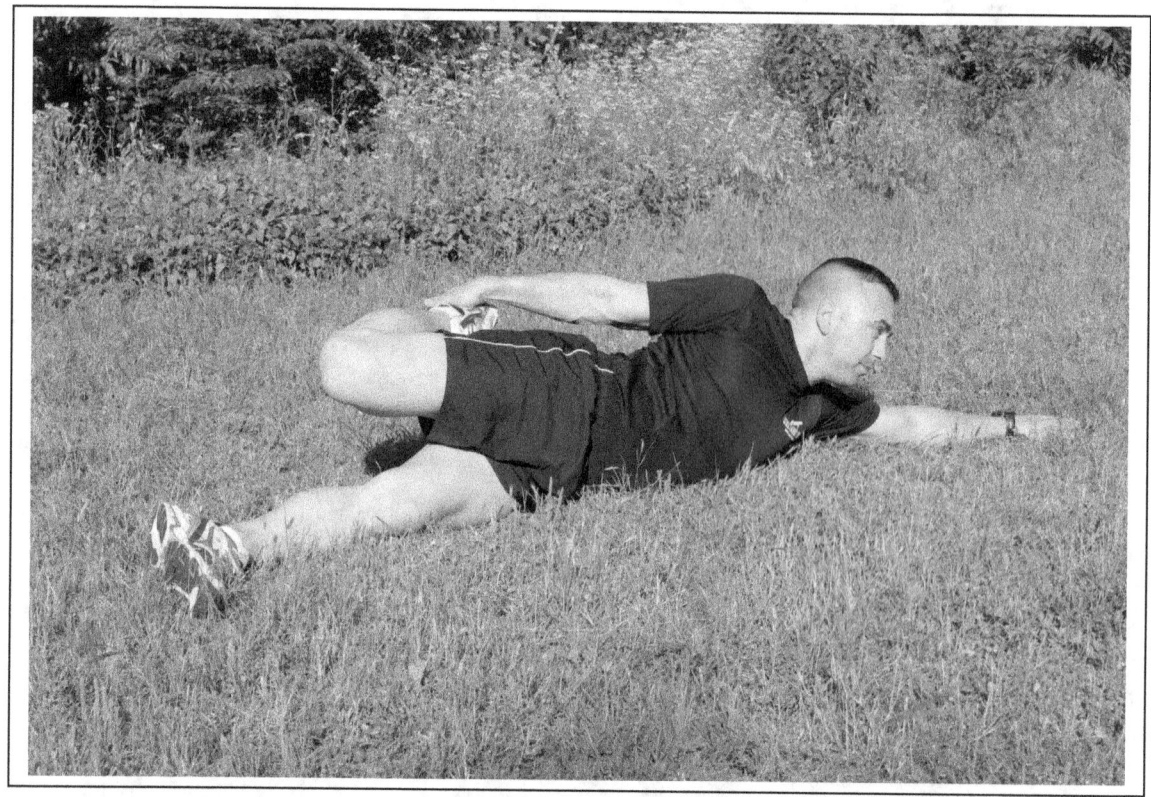

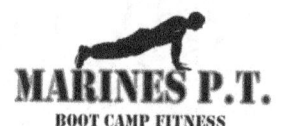

HAMSTRING STRETCH
(Lying down)

This is another hamstring stretch you can use. The hamstring is probably one of the most pulled muscles during exercises, so make sure you stretch this muscle well. Lying on your back, lift your right leg and pull it back. Make sure you grasp your leg just behind the knee as shown. Try to keep your knee as straight as possible.

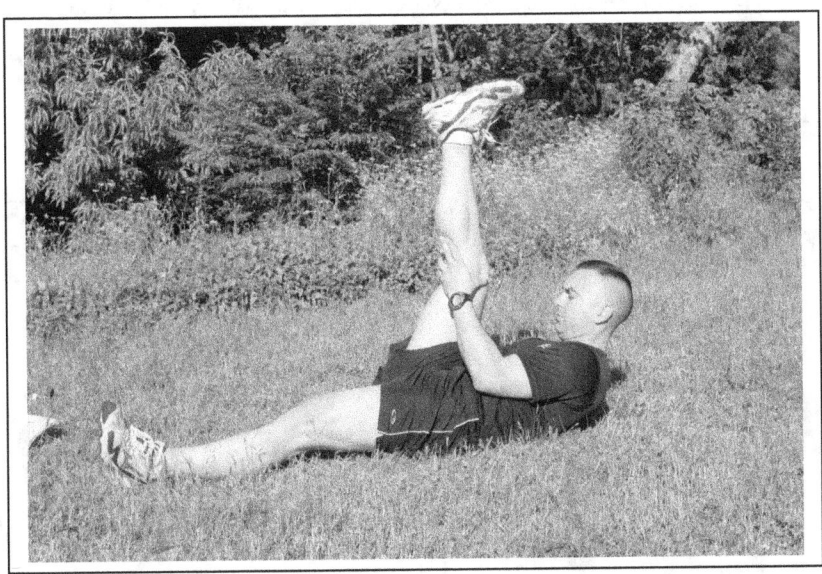

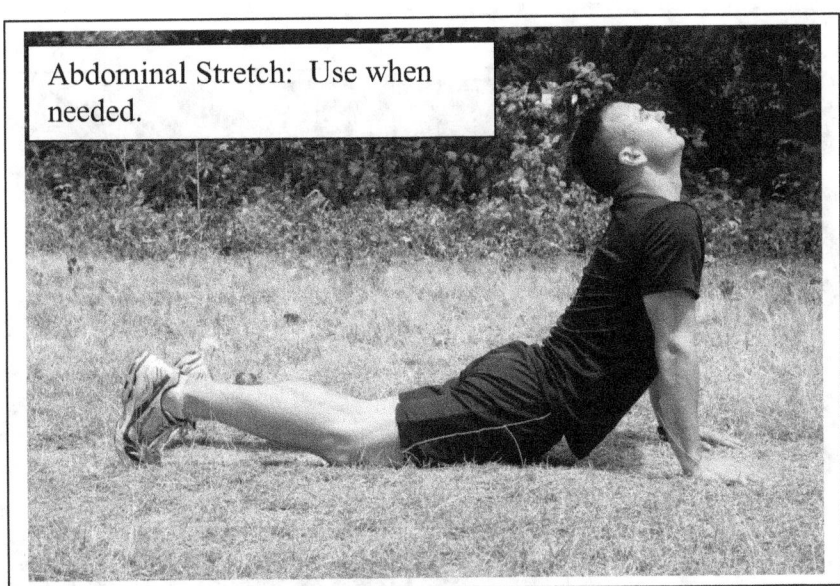

Abdominal Stretch: Use when needed.

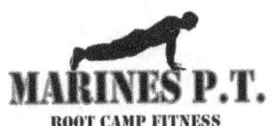

MARINES P.T.
BOOT CAMP FITNESS

EXERCISE DEMO PHOTOS

PUSH-UPS

Start in the up position. Back straight! No sagging or sticking your rear in the air. While looking forward go down until your back and elbows are even as shown. The count at the bottom is 1, when you come back up that is 2 and back down for 3 and up again for the end of your 4 count push-up. Repeat many times! (Note: You may use your knees if needed)

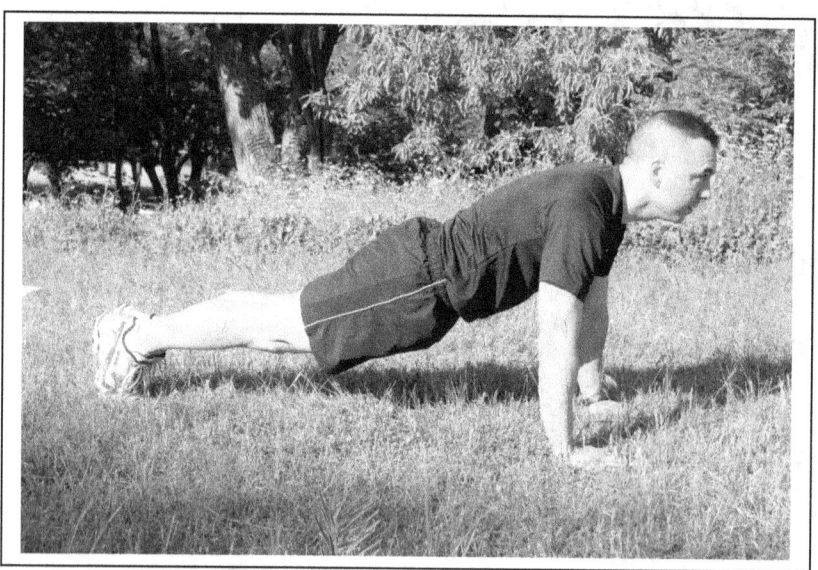

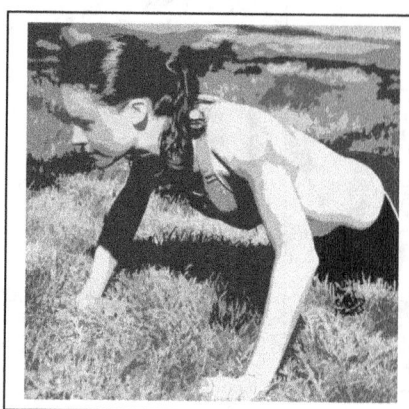

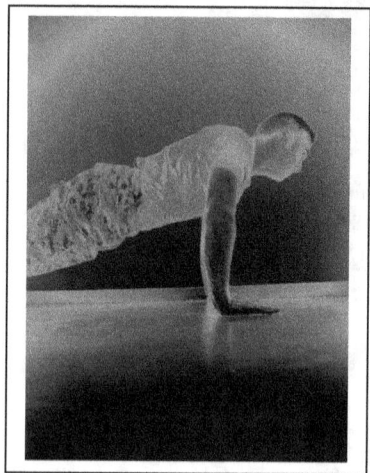

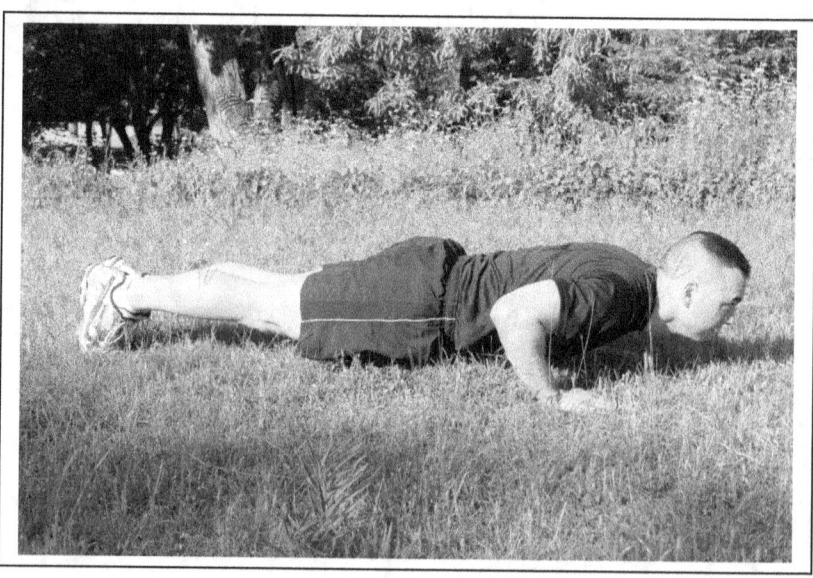

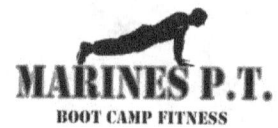

MARINES P.T.
BOOT CAMP FITNESS

SIDE STRADDLE HOPS
(A Fancy name for jumping jacks)

Start with your feet together and arms straight down at your sides as shown. As you jump up raise your arms over your head and spread your legs then land with your legs spread and arms over your head. On your second jump, bring your hands down and legs back together just like you started.

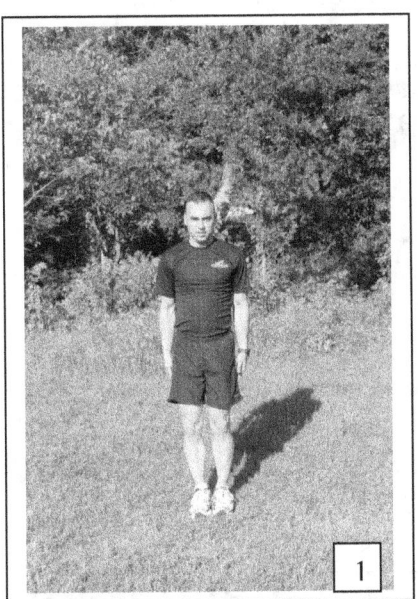
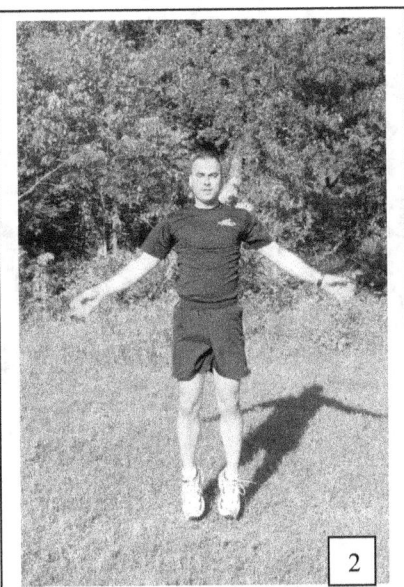
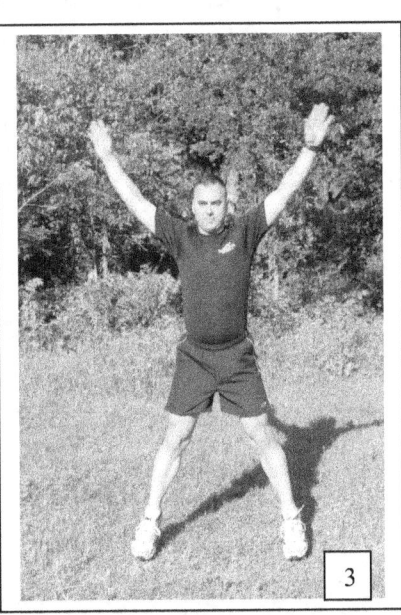

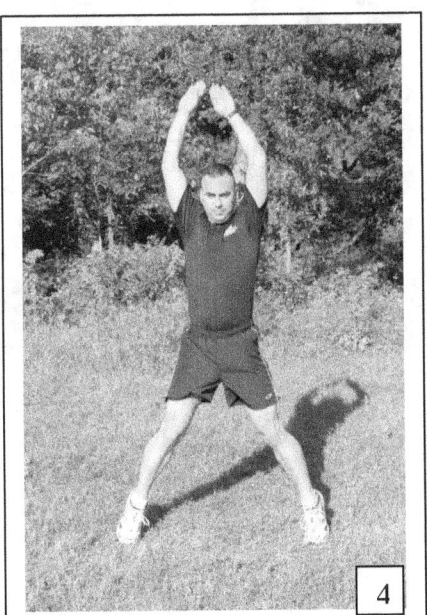
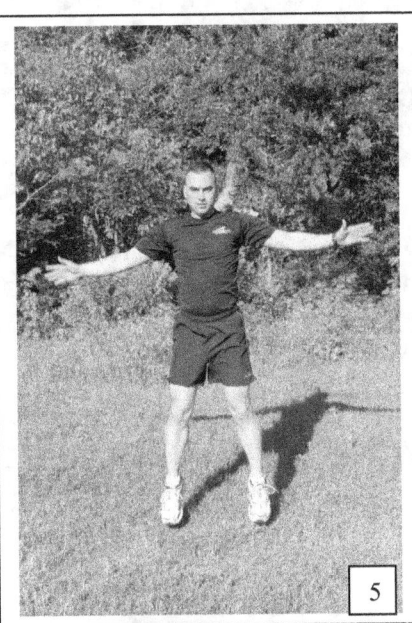
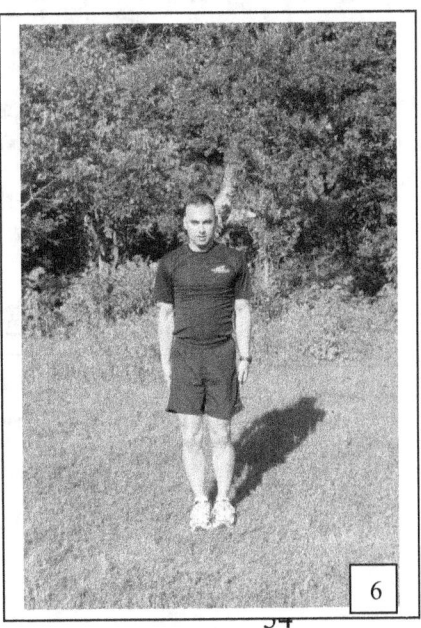

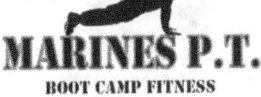

MARINES P.T.
BOOT CAMP FITNESS

DIVE BOMBERS

These is a quite difficult exercise to learn and complete. Your starting position is just like a regular push-up except your rear is in the air as shown. You then go down like a pushup, then push forward like a snake for a count of 1 as shown. Make sure you do not touch the ground with your chest, or any part of your legs. No cheating. Then you reverse the process going back, then push yourself back up for a count of 2. Repeat this process for the counts 3 and 4 and you have just completed 1 four count Dive Bomber push-up. When you can do 20 of these 4 count dive bomber pushups in perfect form, send me an e-mail to marinespt@gmail.com. I want proof!

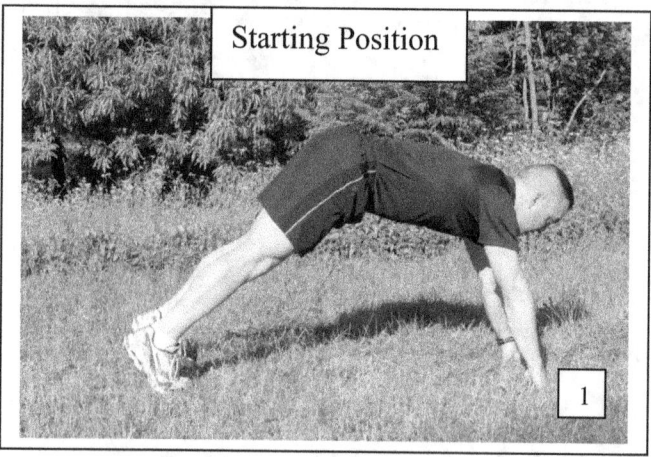

Starting Position

1

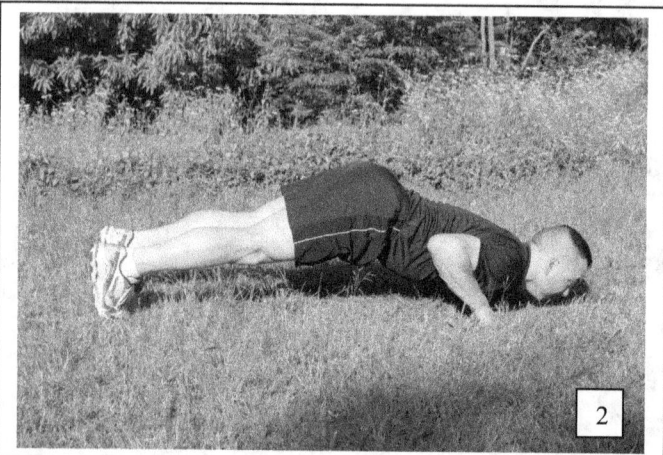

2

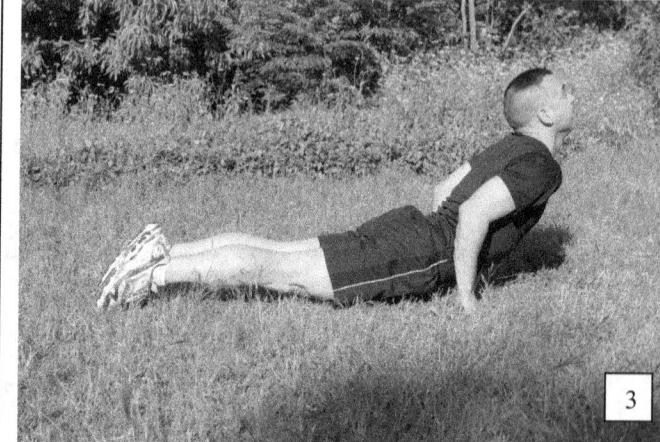

3

The top photo 1 is the start. Photo 2 & 3 combined are one count in the 4 count process. Reverse the process and go from photo 3 position back to photo 2 and back to the starting position for count number 2. You should look like a rocking chair.

35

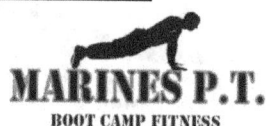

MARINES P.T.
BOOT CAMP FITNESS

SIDE CRUNCHES

Lying on your left side, place your right hand along your side as shown, and your left hand can reach up and grab your right shoulder. Now lift your feet and left shoulder upward at the same time and slide your right hand toward your knee. Repeat on the other side. Each time you come upward is 1 count. You should complete these in 4 counts.

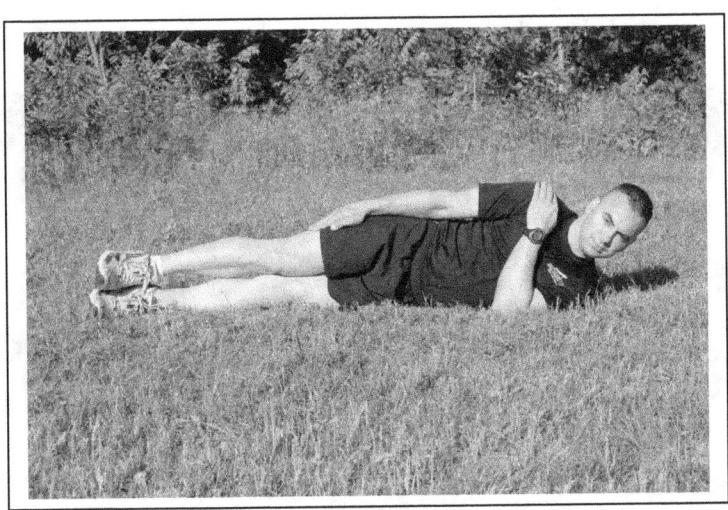

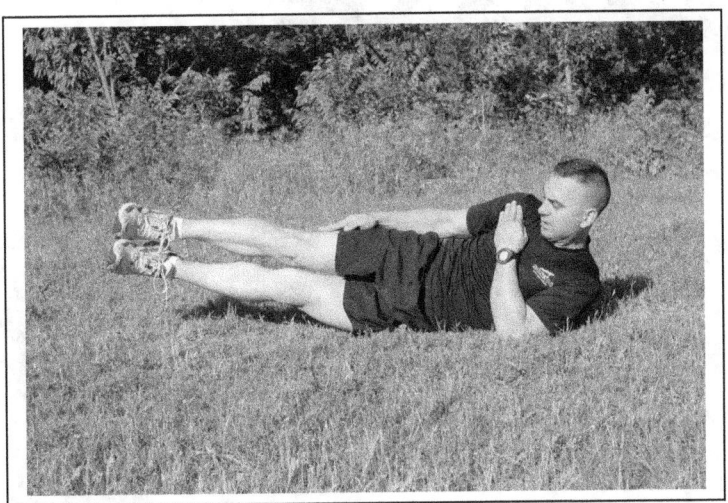

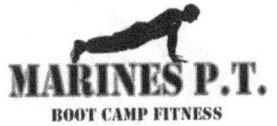

FLUTTER KICKS

Lying on your back, place your hands under your buttocks. You start by lifting your feet 6 inches off the ground while keeping your legs straight and knees locked. Point your toes to help keep your legs straight. Then you begin kicking you're your legs up, one leg at a time while keeping them straight. Your legs should come up to just over a 45-degree angle with the ground. Each leg going up is 1 count. These are 4 count exercises.

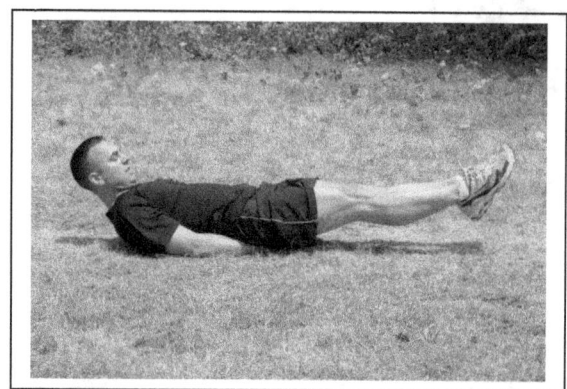
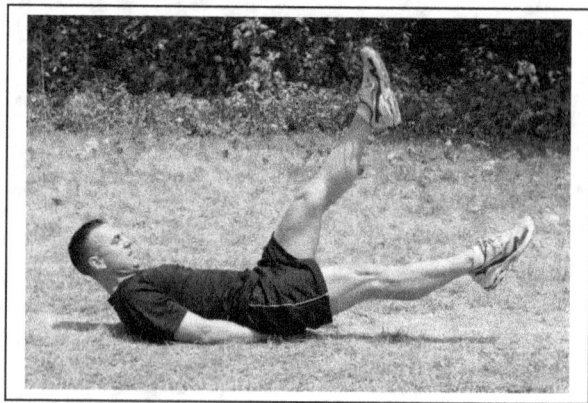

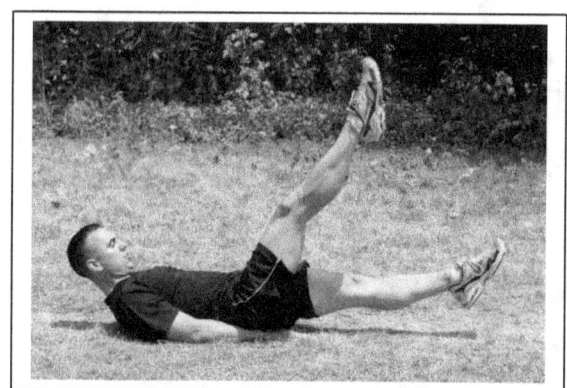

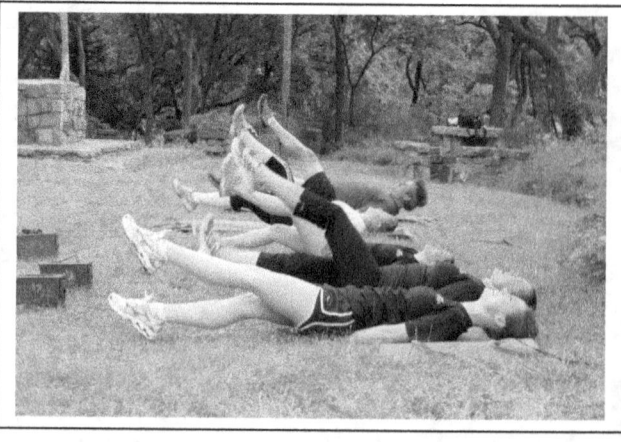

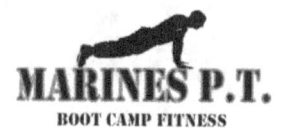

MARINES P.T.
BOOT CAMP FITNESS

DIRTY DOGS

While on all fours raise your right knee up to parallel to the ground as shown.   This exercise should isolate your buttocks. Make sure you don't lean too far to the opposite side so you can ensure you use your buttocks to lift your knee and not your waist. Repeat for left leg. Only do one side at a time.

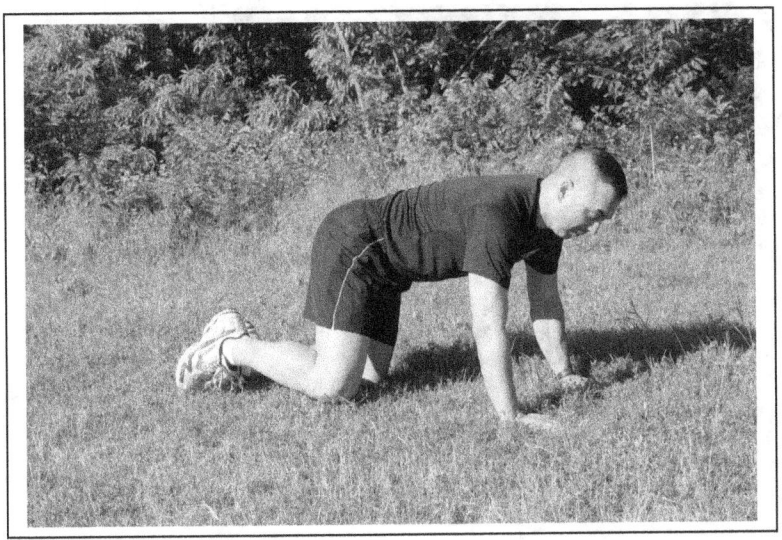

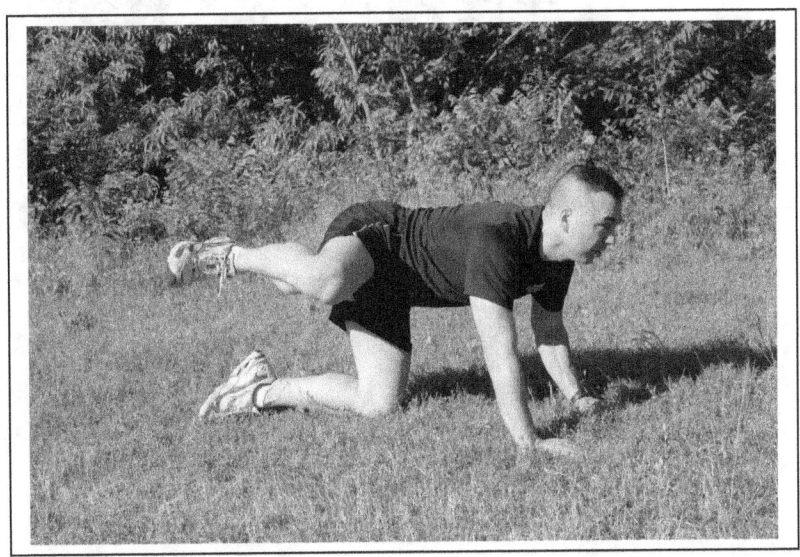

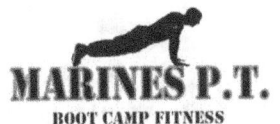

MARINES P.T.
BOOT CAMP FITNESS

DONKEY KICKS

While on all fours, kick your leg out as shown below. Point your toe and keep your leg as straight as possible. You should also kick you leg slightly upward. Repeat for the other leg. Do one side at a time.

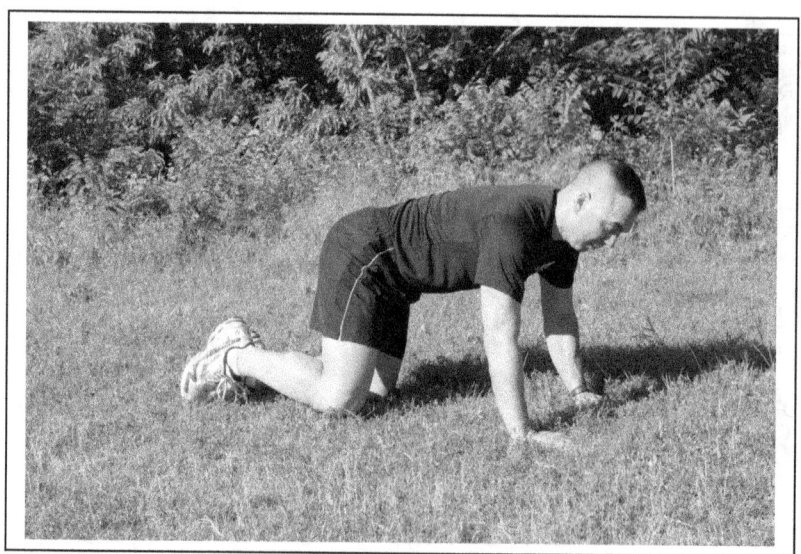

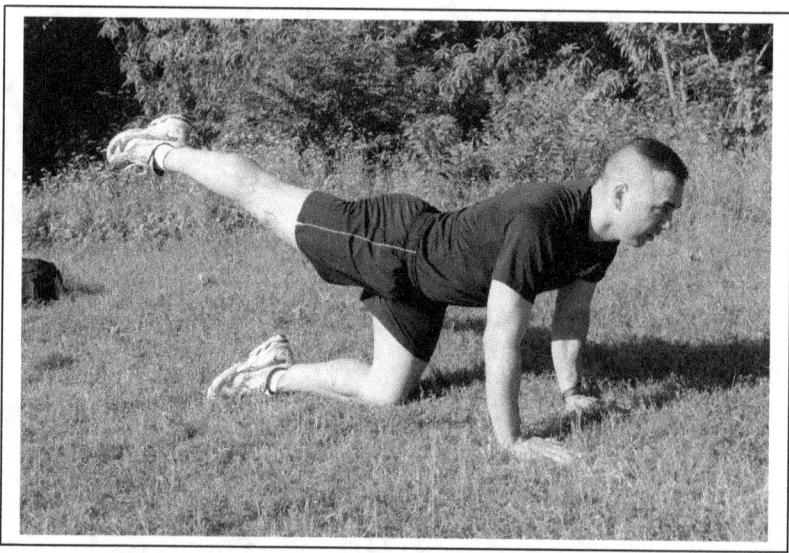

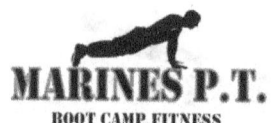

CROSS OVER CRUNCHES
Also called
ELBOW TO KNEE CRUNCHES

Lying on your back as shown, cross your right leg up also as shown. Then begin the exercise doing a crunch and touching your left elbow to your right knee or thigh. Each time you touch your knee or thigh is 1 count. These are done in 4 counts. Do one side, then switch over crossing your left leg over and touch your right elbow to your left knee. You can touch your elbow just below the knee as well.

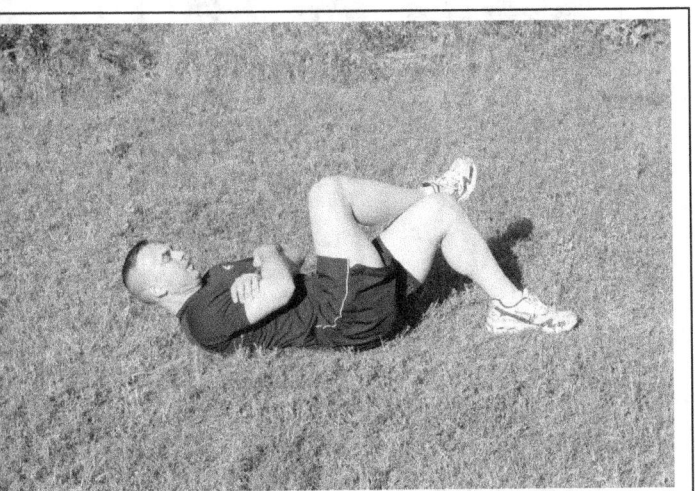
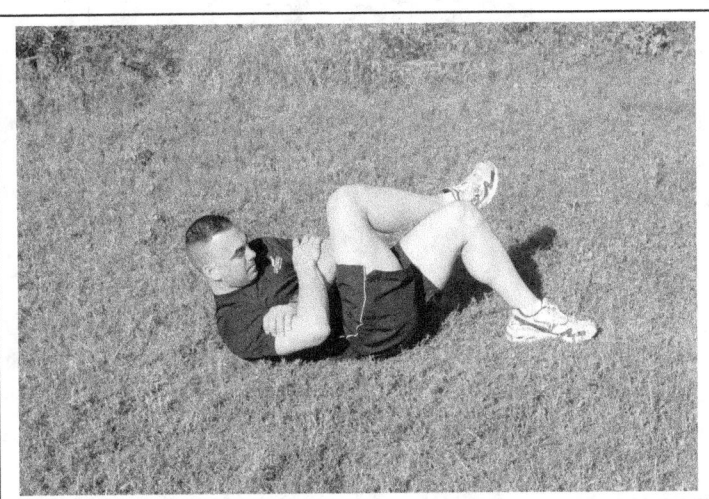

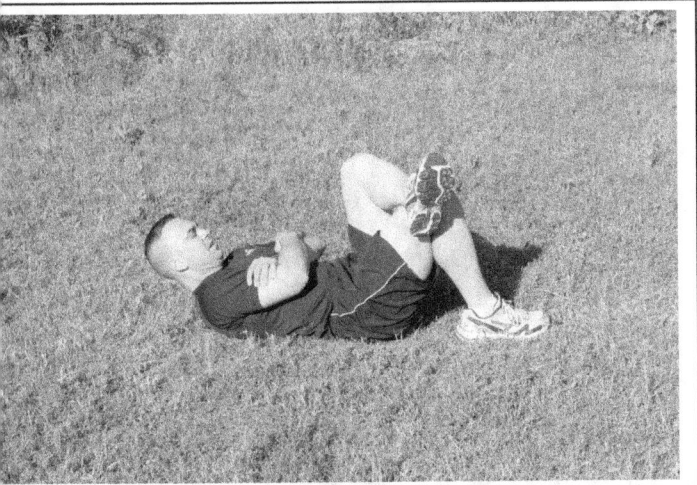
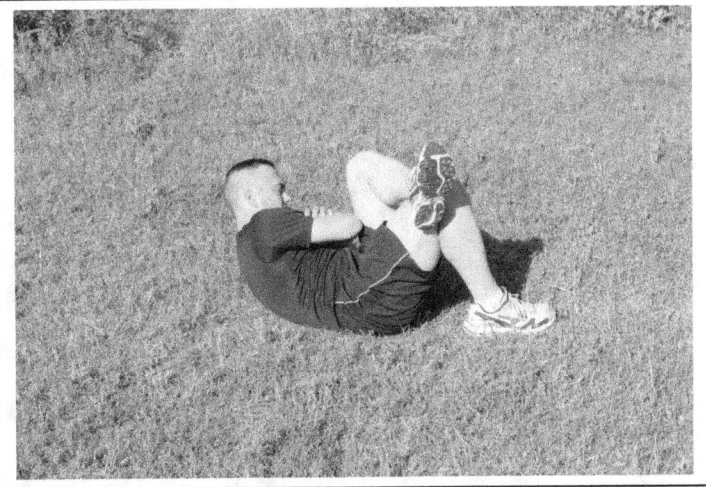

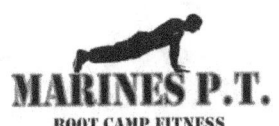

MARINES P.T.
BOOT CAMP FITNESS

STEAM ENGINES

While standing, place your hands behind your head. Lift your left knee as shown and touch your left elbow to your right knee. Continue the exercise with lifting your right knee and touching it with your left elbow in rapid succession. Each touch of the knee is one count.

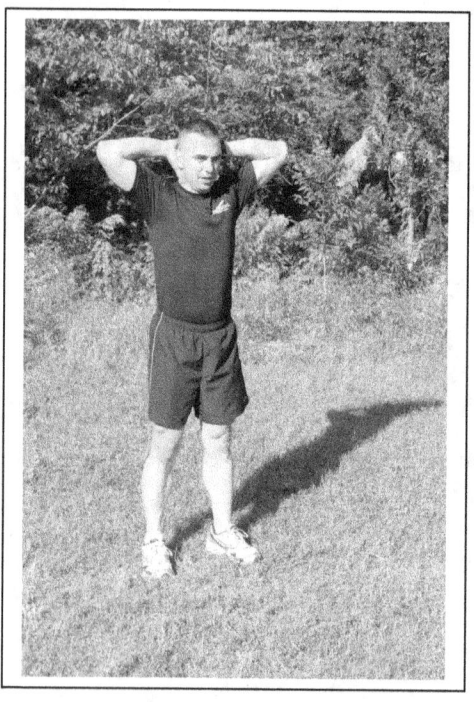 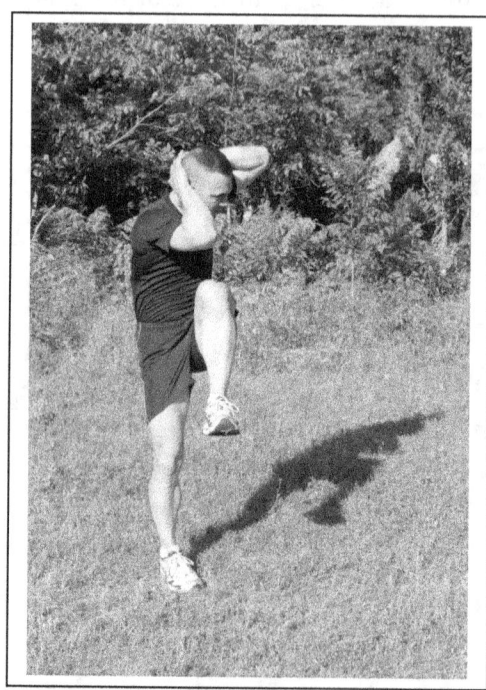

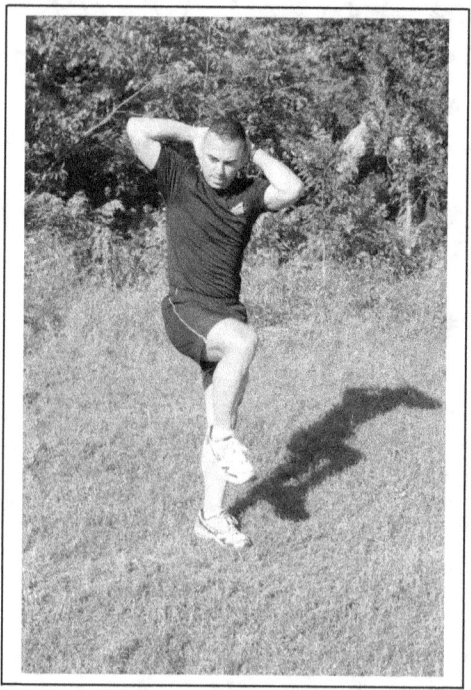 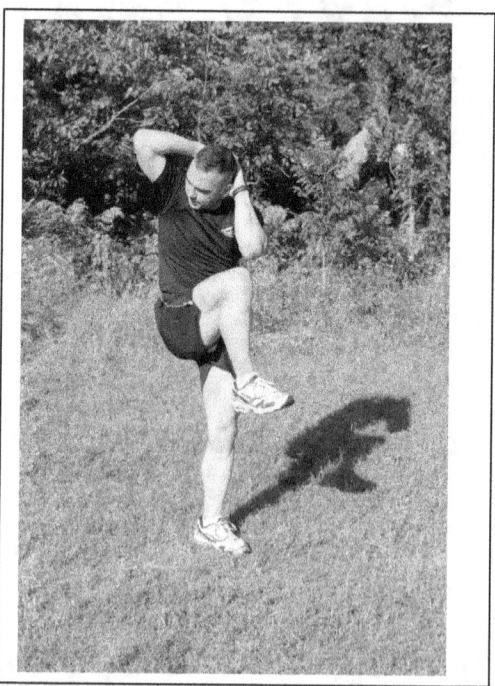

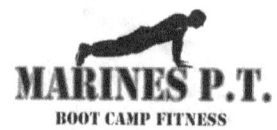

8 COUNT BODY BUILDERS

Begin this exercise with your hands on your hips and feet slightly spread apart as shown. Follow each count for the entire 8-count exercise. All eight counts combined are one repetition. You basically crouch down, kick your legs out, spread your legs, bring them back together, do a push-up, and then get back up. This one may take a few times to get the hang of.

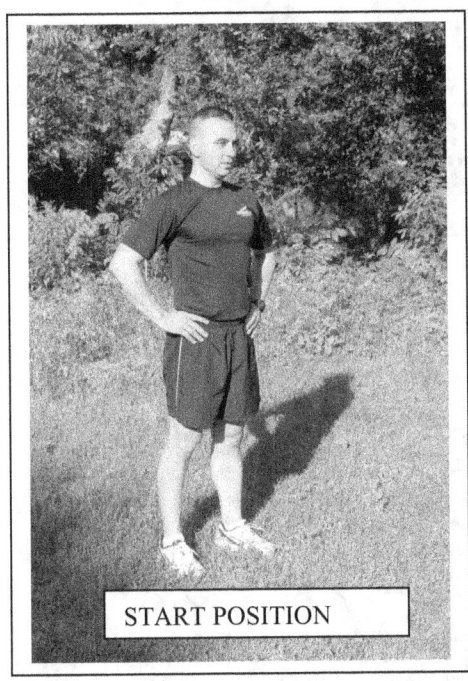

START POSITION

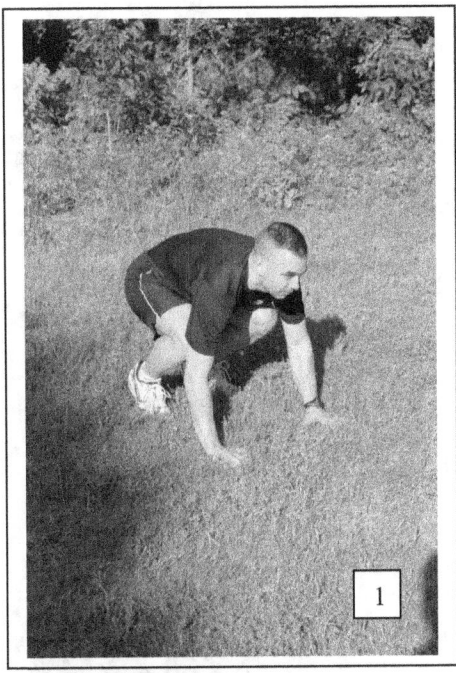

1

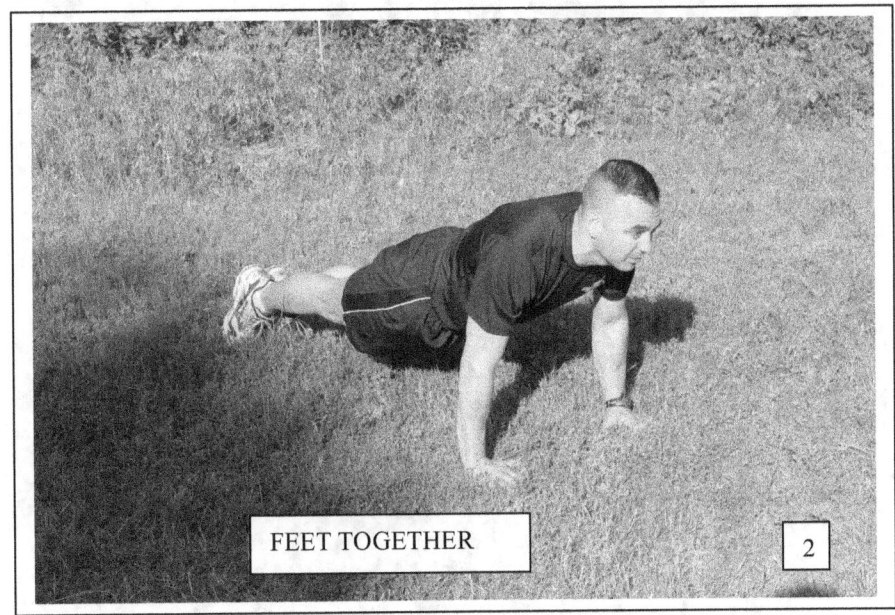

FEET TOGETHER

2

42

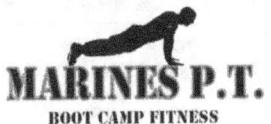

MARINES P.T.
BOOT CAMP FITNESS

8 COUNT BODY BUILDERS

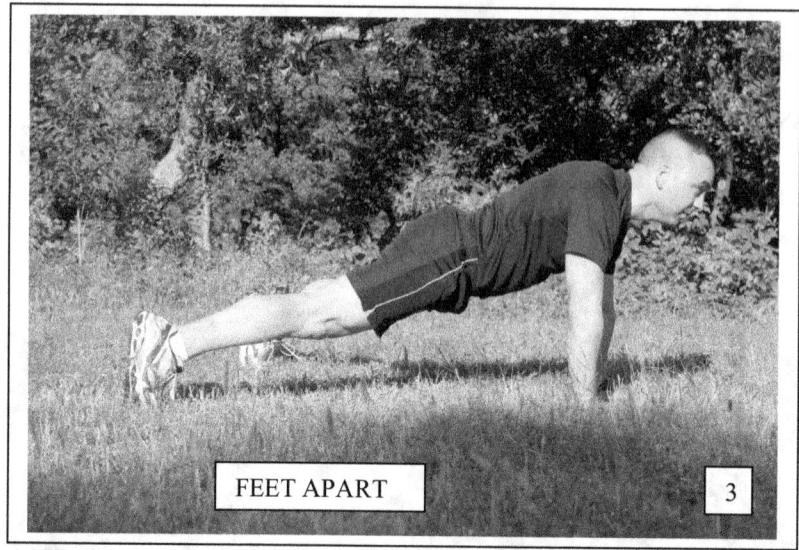

FEET APART

3

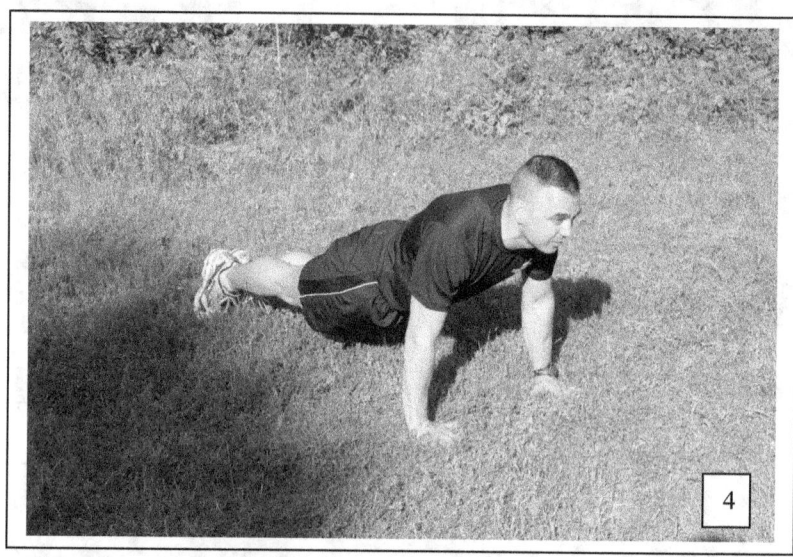

4

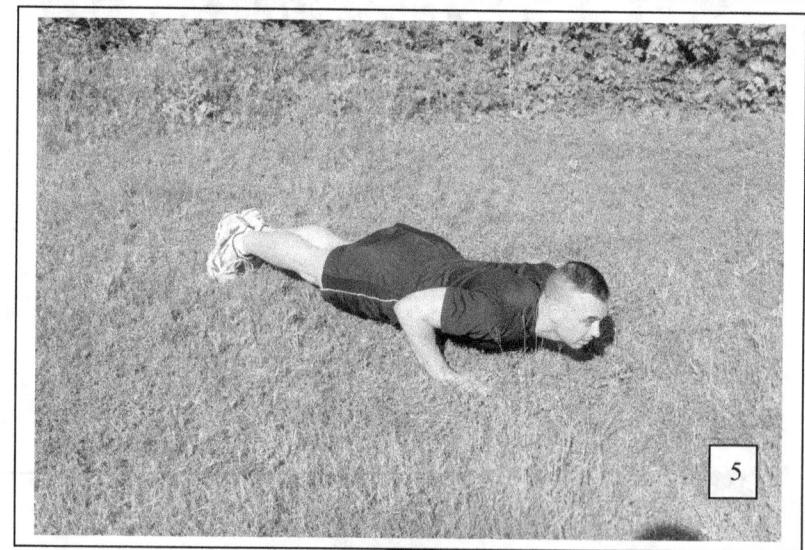

5

MARINES P.T.
BOOT CAMP FITNESS

8 COUNT BODY BUILDERS

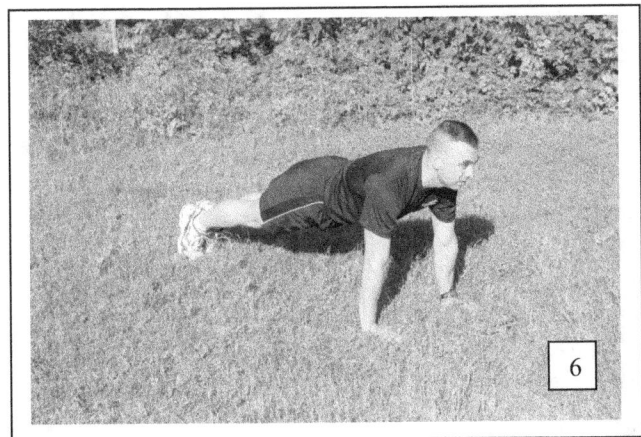

6

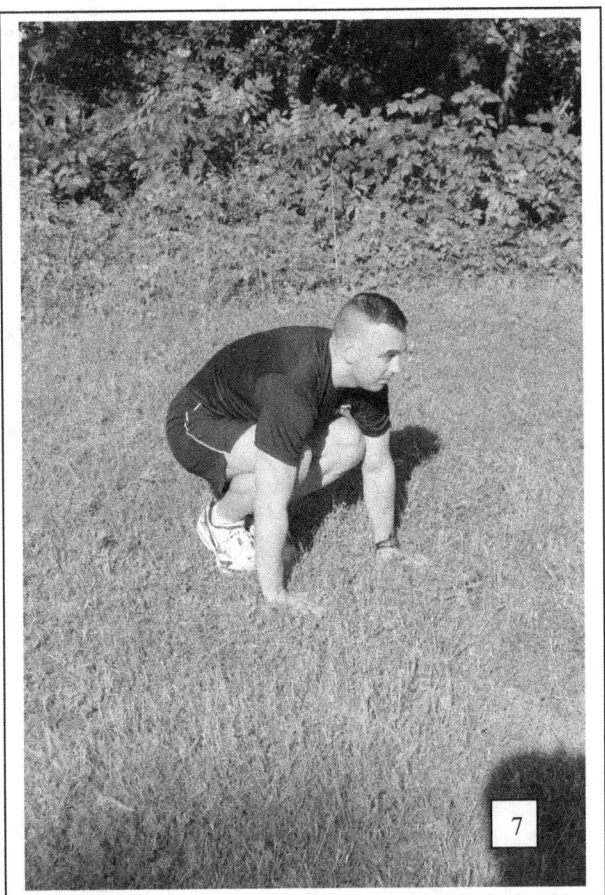

7

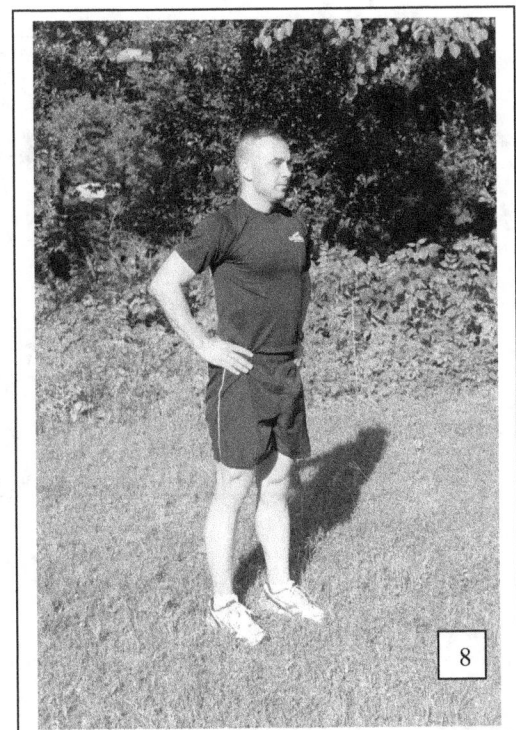

8

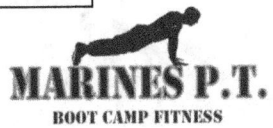

MARINES P.T.
BOOT CAMP FITNESS

WIDE POSITION PUSH-UPS

These pushups are just like regular pushups except you spread your hands further out. This push-up works more of the chest and shoulders and less or your triceps.

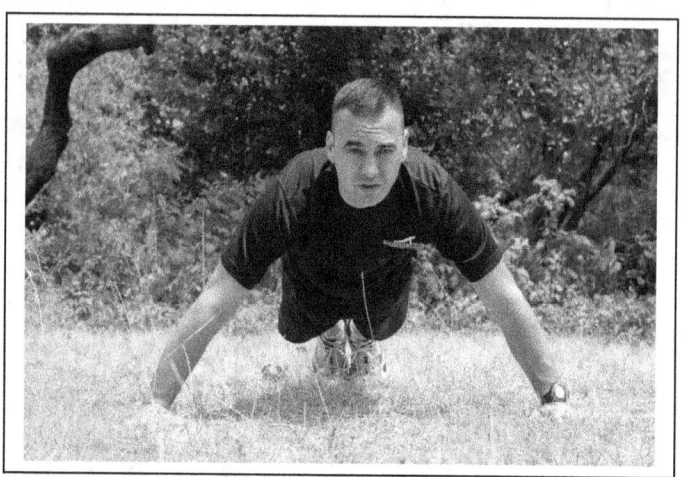

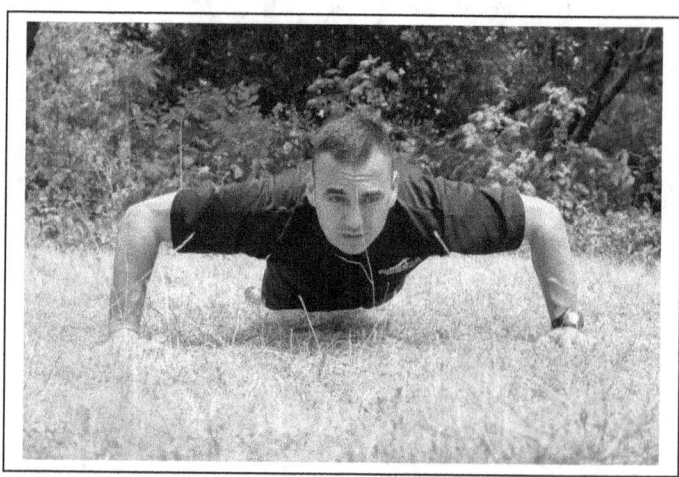

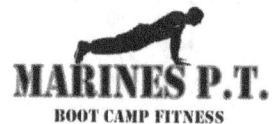

LUNGES

Starting with your left or right leg, take a step forward (not too big, not too small) and go down until your right knee nearly touches the ground. Push back up to the standing position and repeat with your other leg. Going down is count 1, coming back up is count 2, going down with the second leg is count 3, and coming back up is count 4. We use the ammo cans filled with sand while doing our lunges at Marines P.T. Boot Camp Fitness.

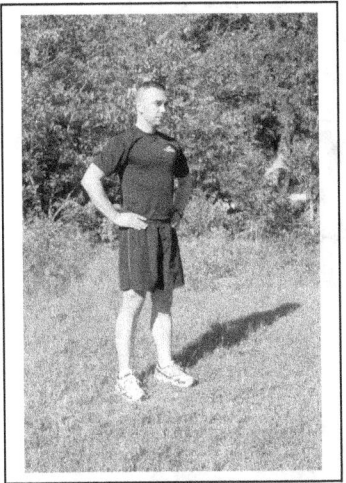
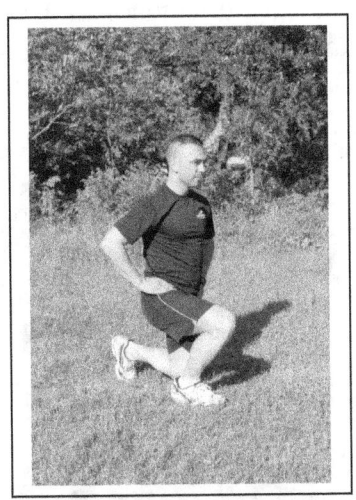
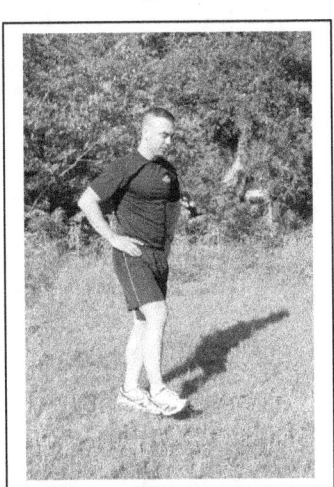

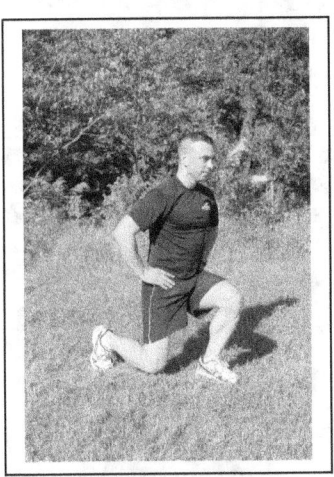
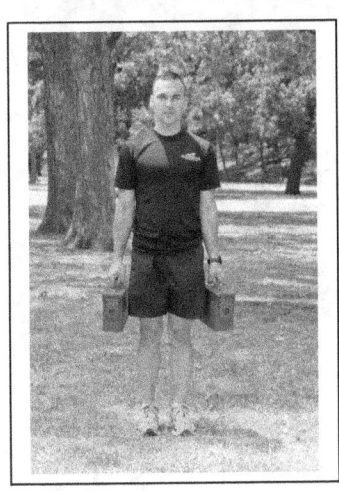
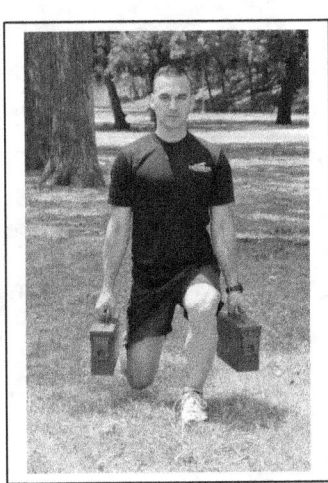

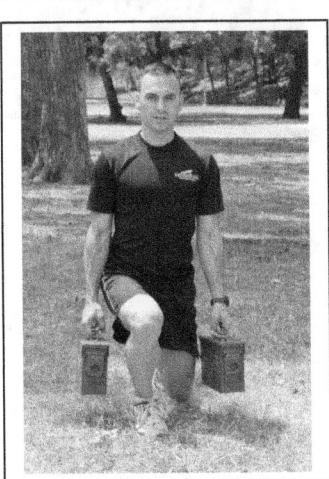

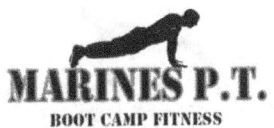

MARINES P.T.
BOOT CAMP FITNESS

46

MOUNTAIN CLIMBERS

Get into the push-up position with your left leg brought forward as shown below for your starting position. Try not to stick your rear too far in the air. The exercises consists of you pumping your legs forward, and extending them all the way back again like you are climbing a mountain. Keep you knees pointed forward and make sure to extend your legs all the way back on each pump. Do not angle your knees and feet outward.

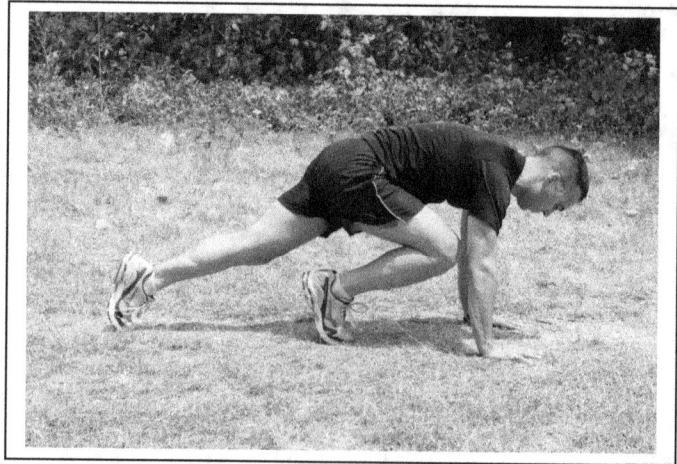

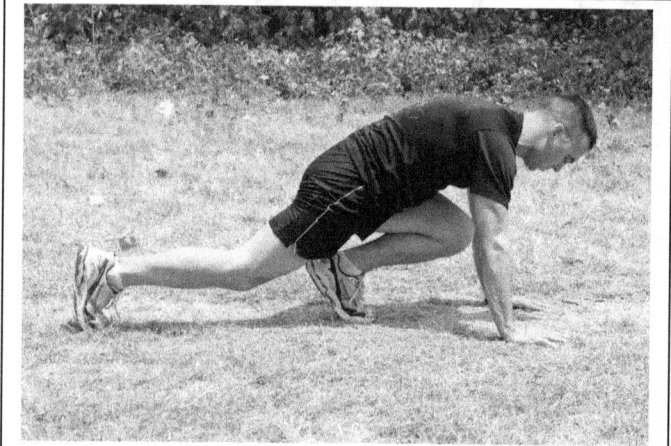

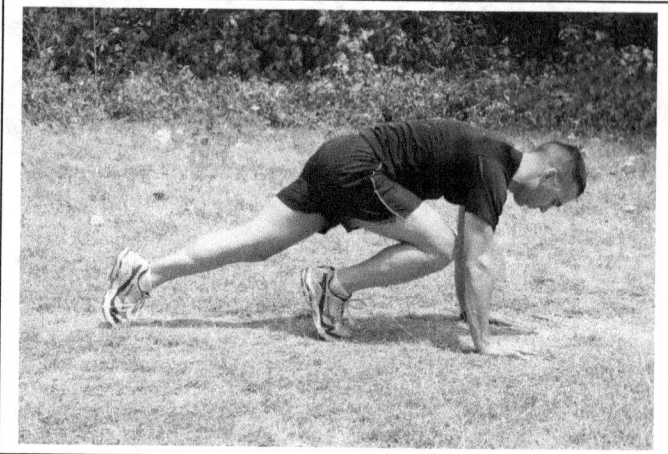

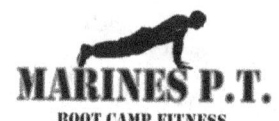

MARINES P.T.
BOOT CAMP FITNESS

CRUNCHES

The crunches I use for my workouts are with both feet in the air and crossed over as shown below. We also do crunches the Marines Corps standard way by having someone hold your feet. In each case you grab your biceps and touch your elbows to your thighs. The bottoms of your shoulder blades must touch the ground for the crunch to count.

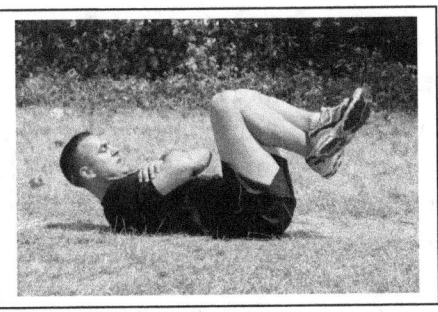 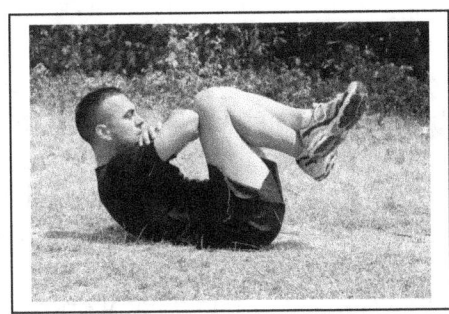

Fitness Test Crunches

These should be done with someone holding your feet for best results. While performing the exercise, your hands should always grasp your biceps, and your elbows must touch your upper thigh to count.

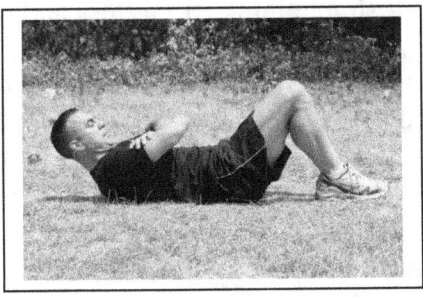 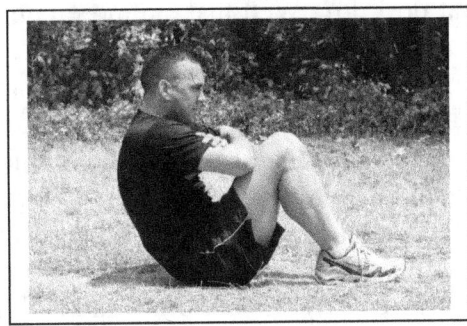

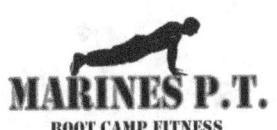

MARINES P.T.
BOOT CAMP FITNESS

PART IV

DIET & NUTRITION

(A very brief note)

My thoughts on Diet and Nutrition are quite simple. Eat less move more! There is no doubt that proper nutrition and diet are an essential part of attaining your personal goals. Without a good nutrition plan you will only go so far in creating a healthy, long-term fitness lifestyle. I will not claim to be an expert in nutrition nor will I claim that I follow the best nutrition plan I can. I do what works for my fitness goals, and me… and that's the key. You need to do what works best for you and your goals. There is a wealth of free information on the internet that could give you much of the info you are looking for free of charge. However, consult your doctor or a nutritionist for the best results.

Many have asked me what I do for nutrition and what I've seen work. First off, the only diet that I have personally witnessed remove 70+ pounds from someone in about 7 months was the Atkins diet. I am only making a statement of fact based on what I have been exposed to. I have not seen every diet, and I'm sure there are diet stories like Jarred from Subway that also work. But the only diet that I have seen with my own two eyes work is the Atkins diet. My parents both went on this diet and I was amazed by what they accomplished 7 months. The only down side to it was that if you stray from the diet you gain it all back quick….and they did.

What do I do? Well that's a more complex but very simple thing. I eat less and move about like a crazy wild man all the time. I simply train a lot and have done an ok job of eating mostly the right stuff. I have nearly eliminated fast food and sodas from my diet in the last 2 years. My nutrition as I look back over the years, was pretty well balanced and not over indulgent. I usually ate a small breakfast like oatmeal or cereal with milk. I skipped lunch for many years or ate a granola bar or some snack, and a great dinner. My dinner was the key for me. I had steak and potatoes, spaghetti with meat sauce, tuna casserole, pork chops and biscuits. Come to think of it…I eat pretty good. Now some of you may be saying, "but I though breakfast was the most important meal" maybe it is for some people….it just wasn't for me. Remember, I over compensate with large amounts of exercise. I think for the most part I have been lucky. I think my being extremely active since birth has been my saving grace. I can't say that I have always made nutrition a focus I it is becoming more so as I grow older. So in closing on the diet and nutrition side of things, find a long-term solution that works for you and your goals. Find something you plan to stick with and make part of your lifestyle.

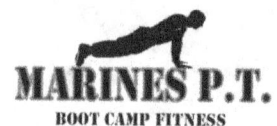

CLOSING

We are defined by what we do when nobody is looking.

We create our lifestyle by what activities we choose to partake in, and much of what we do will go unnoticed in the moment, but noticed over time in your appearance and personality. Both good deeds and weak moments can pass without a witness to be found.

- Will you eat ice cream or drink a glass of orange juice?

- Will you actually jog that mile or walk it and tell your friends you ran it?

Nobody is looking. There are no shortcuts in fitness or anything else for that matter. So take personal responsibility for what you do when no one is around and reap the benefits later. After years of leadership in the U.S. Marines and the corporate world, I have discovered a very important fact. **"<u>No amount of motivation and coercion on my part will ever substitute for personal drive and effort on your part.</u> "**

Take this workout book and use it to build your body and mind. Use it to make new friends. Start your own fitness group and enjoy the camaraderie it brings. Good luck, God speed, and remain Semper Fidelis.

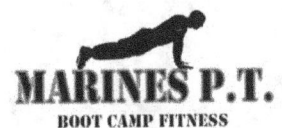

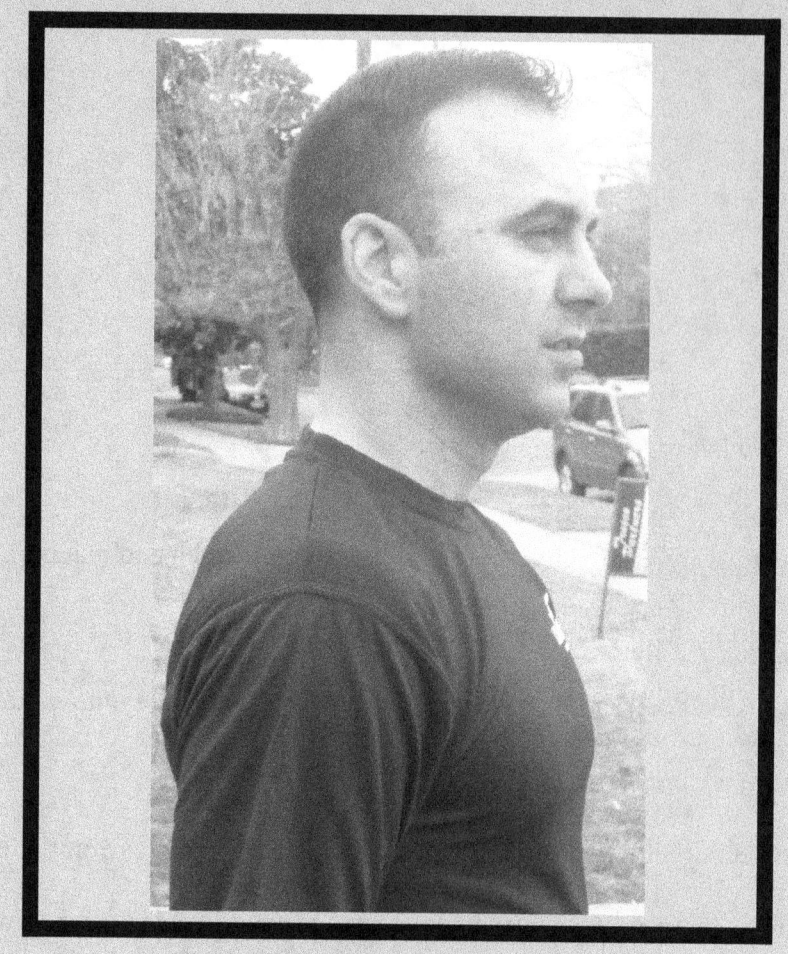

" If you want to get in shape quickly and are willing to work hard, this is the class for you. "
-Jean

" great way to get outside and get some healthy training, meet new people and have fun while working out. "
-Christianne

" This is a GREAT way to get into shape! While the exercises are based on the military, you're not treated like you're in the military. ... "
-Patsy Caldwell

" I joined *Marines PT* to loose weight for my wedding and within a few months I had lost inches on my waist, legs and buttocks. I fit into pants I had not fit into since college!!!! I am well on my way to looking great for my wedding and it is all thanks to this boot camp! My fiance loves it!"
-Erin

I have been with Marines P.T. now for about 5 months, and I can honestly say that within 2 1/2 months I found a drop in my waistline! I went down 1 1/2 SIZES only doing Marines P.T. Workouts 3 days a week…. a THANK YOU is long overdue!
-Libby

www.ingramcontent.com/pod-product-compliance
Lightning Source LLC
Chambersburg PA
CBHW081002290526
45795CB00009B/3051